Boosting Your Metabolism

FOR DUMMIES®

A Wiley Brand

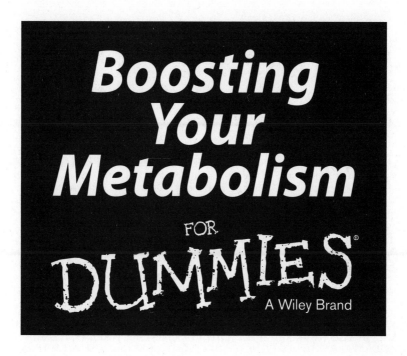

Boosting Your Metabolism

FOR DUMMIES®

A Wiley Brand

by Rachel Berman, R.D.

Director of Nutrition, CalorieCount.com

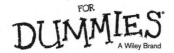

FOR DUMMIES®
A Wiley Brand

Boosting Your Metabolism For Dummies®

Published by
John Wiley & Sons, Inc.
111 River St.
Hoboken, NJ 07030-5774
www.wiley.com

For general information on our other products and services, please contact our Customer Care Department within the U.S. at 877-762-2974, outside the U.S. at 317-572-3993, or fax 317-572-4002.

For technical support, please visit www.wiley.com/techsupport.

Wiley publishes in a variety of print and electronic formats and by print-on-demand. Some material included with standard print versions of this book may not be included in e-books or in print-on-demand. If this book refers to media such as a CD or DVD that is not included in the version you purchased, you may download this material at http://booksupport.wiley.com. For more information about Wiley products, visit www.wiley.com.

Library of Congress Control Number: 2013933957

ISBN 978-1-118-49157-7 (pbk); ISBN 978-1-118-50177-1 (ePub); ISBN 978-1-118-50184-9 (ePDF); ISBN 978-1-118-50186-3 (eMobi)

Manufactured in the United States of America

10 9 8 7 6 5 4 3 2 1

About the Author

Rachel Berman, R.D., C.D./N. is a registered dietitian who has helped thousands of clients lose weight and improve their health. She's worked in hospitals, clinics, and online to translate scientific information into practical advice for various patient populations. Berman's philosophy emphasizes balance and moderation, and she's passionate about helping others develop a healthier relationship with food.

Currently, Berman is the Director of Nutrition for CalorieCount.com, a free wellness website with more than 5 million members. She manages nutrition-related content and helps develop tools for the website and its mobile apps. In 2011, Berman spearheaded a service for Calorie Count members to receive personalized online health coaching from registered dietitians.

Berman is a nationally recognized expert and has been featured in publications such as the *Huffington Post, Us* magazine, the *Chicago Tribune,* FOX Business Online, and *Shape* magazine. She has also appeared on *The Today Show* and various local television and radio health segments.

Berman earned her B.S. in Nutritional Sciences from Cornell University and completed her dietetic internship with the North Shore-LIJ Health Care System. She is recognized by the Academy of Nutrition and Dietetics as a registered dietitian. Berman is passionate about trying new foods, restaurants, and exercise classes. She lives in New York City.

Author's Acknowledgments

I'm so grateful to the team at Wiley Publishing for making this an experience of a lifetime. A big thank you to Tracy Boggier, my acquisitions editor, for your incredible encouragement throughout the entire process and convincing me that yes, I can write a book! My project editor, Corbin Collins, kept me on my toes and truly provided me with all the support I needed to complete this project. Thank you to my technical editor, Susan Male Smith, for your attention to detail to enhance the scientific accuracy and completeness of this book. And to Emily Nolan, for testing out all of the recipes and making tweaks to ensure they are both nutritious and delicious.

Thank you to my fitness guru Kimberly Fleming and psychology expert Dr. Sarah Parker for letting me consult you on aspects that are not my primary areas of expertise. Your knowledge helped me ensure this book is current with the latest research and trends in those areas. Thank you also to stellar dietetic students Leyla Shamayeva and Lauren Borg for your valuable research assistance. A special thanks to the folks over at CalorieCount.com, specifically Igor Lebovic and Howard Sherman, for fully backing my decision to write this book while juggling my full time job. I couldn't have done this without your support.

From the bottom of my heart, thank you to all of my family and friends for your love and encouragement. I'm grateful to my parents for their undying support: Mom, for having the foresight to send me to a nutritionist as a teen, which opened my eyes to the field, and Dad, for imparting decades of knowledge about the media and book-writing process. Thank you, Marc, for being a constant reminder that "Everything is going to be okay"!

Last but not least, I'd like to express my gratitude to all of my clients along the way and, especially, to the readers of this book. Thank you for wanting to know the truth about how to boost your metabolism so that you can live a healthy, balanced life!

Publisher's Acknowledgments

We're proud of this book; please send us your comments at http://dummies.custhelp.com. For other comments, please contact our Customer Care Department within the U.S. at 877-762-2974, outside the U.S. at 317-572-3993, or fax 317-572-4002.

Some of the people who helped bring this book to market include the following:

Acquisitions, Editorial, and Vertical Websites

Editor: Corbin Collins

Acquisitions Editor: Tracy Boggier

Assistant Editor: David Lutton

Editorial Program Coordinator: Joe Niesen

Technical Editor: Susan Male Smith

Recipe Tester: Emily Nolan

Senior Editorial Manager: Jennifer Ehrlich

Editorial Manager: Carmen Krikorian

Editorial Assistant: Rachelle Amick

Art Coordinator: Alicia B. South

Composition Services

Project Coordinator: Katherine Crocker

Layout and Graphics: Jennifer Creasey, Joyce Haughey

Proofreaders: Melissa Cossell, Susan Moritz, Lisa Young Stiers

Indexer: Riverside Indexes, Inc.

Special Art: Kathryn Born

Photographers: Matt Bowen, Bob McNamara

Publishing and Editorial for Consumer Dummies

> **Kathleen Nebenhaus,** Vice President and Executive Publisher

> **David Palmer,** Associate Publisher

> **Kristin Ferguson-Wagstaffe,** Product Development Director

Publishing for Technology Dummies

> **Andy Cummings,** Vice President and Publisher

Composition Services

> **Debbie Stailey,** Director of Composition Services

Contents at a Glance

Table of Contents

Introduction

Welcome to *Boosting Your Metabolism For Dummies!* Whether you've picked up this book because you're tired of a lifetime of dieting or you're making healthy changes for the first time, you're in good hands. You may think that your metabolism is beyond saving, but I assure you that you can take steps to boost your metabolic rate no matter what's going on with you today or what's happened in the past. When you want to lose weight, you typically associate it with restriction, whether that means switching to eating salads and "rabbit food" or becoming a workout-aholic. Although you'll certainly be making changes, you'll find no boot camp in these pages.

For healthy changes to last a lifetime, they have to be realistic for you. Feeling deprived or bored with what you eat and how you move, is no way to live. If you go that route, you'll soon fall into old habits — as I'm sure you've already found out. Instead, this book is an opportunity for you to change the way you think and develop a healthier relationship with yourself so that you can lose weight once and for all.

In this book, I give you easy ways to change the way you eat with meal plans, recipes, and realistic tips to develop new, healthy habits. I show how you can shop, stock up, and eat out, all while making the best food choices. Because exercise is a major part of the equation, I offer workout plans and activities that you can incorporate no matter your fitness level. You definitely don't have to be a professional cook or athlete to make these tips work for you.

I also provide practical advice about sticking to healthy habits within your financial budget and time constraints. A key focus of this book is on the behavioral and mental changes you need to address, which are typically missing from traditional diet books. You may know *what* changes you need to make, but not *how* to make them last. It's the *how* that's the essence of a lifestyle change.

About This Book

I've organized things here so that you'll easily find the information you need to start taking steps to boost your metabolism today. I won't be offended if you don't read every word, and you definitely don't need to memorize anything to move on to the next section. In fact, this book isn't meant to be read cover to cover. I encourage you to feel free to skip around to the sections that are most relevant for you and your life.

You might start by taking a look at the table of contents to see what catches your eye. If this is your first nutrition book, or to brush up on the science behind nutrition, start with Chapter 1 to learn all about the basics of metabolism. If you're heading to the grocery store to start cooking, check out Chapters 7–10 for recipe ideas or Chapter 5 for the must-buys. Or start flipping through, saying, "Eeny, meeny, miny, moe," put your finger down on a page, and read it if a heading catches your interest. I wrote this for all who are trying to improve their metabolic profile — whether you're young or further along in years, male or female, athlete or couch potato.

Conventions Used in This Book

My mission is for you to easily grasp and apply the information in this book to your everyday life. Therefore, I use conventions to make the info as smooth and easy to get through as possible.

- ✔ I provide a lot of content in flexible terms with alternate options. I don't expect you to follow the sample meal plans or workouts to a tee. You can follow the guidelines and fit in the specific foods or exercises that are realistic for you.

- ✔ I write in layman's terms as much as possible, without too much science-y mumbo jumbo. If you're a science nerd like me, though, don't worry — there's plenty of science here, but it's described in easy-to-understand language.

- ✔ I frequently put quotations around the word "diet" or words like "good" and "bad" when talking about certain foods or habits. This indicates that I don't buy into common definitions of these words and want to redefine them for you. For example, "dieting" is typically associated with restriction or the fad of the week, whereas the true definition of *diet* really just means what you are eating on a regular basis.

- ✔ In the exercise section, I often provide more than one photo so that you can see the progression of the exercise from start to finish.

- ✔ Whenever I refer to a web address for additional information, it will appear in monotype font `which looks like this` so that it stands out.

- ✔ When this book was printed, some web addresses may have needed to break across two lines of text. If that happened, rest assured that there are no extra characters (such as hyphens) to indicate the break. Just type in exactly what you see in this book, pretending the line break doesn't exist.

✔ The recipes can be tweaked to meet your specific needs. If you don't like nuts, for example, then you don't have to eat them or include them in the recipe (and if you have an allergy, definitely steer clear!). Swap out what you need and feel free to experiment. None of the recipes is so complicated that you'll mess up the basic properties of cooking. On the recipes, bear in mind the following:

- All temperature degrees are in Fahrenheit.

- All beans can be canned (rinsed and drained) or cooked from dried.

- When I refer to low-fat milk or cheese, you can choose fat-free or 1 percent milkfat.

What You're Not to Read

I mean, you can if you want to, but it's not necessary for you to read anything preceded by the Technical Stuff icon.

Like this.

Because the subject at hand is intertwined with biology, when you see this icon it means what I'm talking about is very science-y, and you can skip it without missing out too much on the larger topic at hand.

It's also not mandatory for you to read the sidebars but if you find your eyes wandering over to one, and the header is appealing to you, that info will just broaden the scope of your understanding even further. Finally, you don't need to read the recipes all the way through — just pick and choose the ones that speak to your taste buds.

Foolish Assumptions

Since you made a foolish assumption that I actually know what I'm talking about by buying this book, I'm going to let you in on some assumptions I made about you while writing this book:

✔ You want to lose weight and make a lifestyle change while doing it. If you don't want to lose weight, you can still learn about the inner workings of metabolism with this book, but the focus is on weight loss.

✔ That it's possible you want a quick fix like you may have tried in the past. I spend the book providing evidence that "quick fixes" are bad for your metabolic rate and discuss how to break out of the dieting mentality for your long-term health.

✔ That you could use a refresher on the ABCs of nutrition, but also are educated enough to understand some of the more complex aspects which affect your metabolism.

How This Book Is Organized

This book divides its chapters into five parts. I cross-reference a lot, so if you want more info on a topic, instead of me repeating it over and over, you can just flip to another chapter or part. I also refer to online content I've written for even more helpful tips and advice in certain areas of interest.

Part 1: Getting Started with Boosting Your Metabolism

With all the myths about metabolism floating around the media and in your social circle, this part gives you a solid footing to be able to wow your friends and amaze yourself with the truth. You'll understand exactly what metabolism is and why you should want to improve it. I go into the factors that impact your metabolic rate and how you can measure your metabolism.

Part II: Laying the Groundwork for Boosting Your Metabolism

Before making any lifestyle change, you've got to take steps to prepare both mentally and physically. In this part, you'll discover how to find the right motivation to last a lifetime. Once you have the mental component down, the behaviors you need to change will come more easily — from the foods you should be cutting down on to those you need to add to boost your metabolic rate. In addition, you get the low-down on the best combinations of foods, optimal meal timing, and flexible sample meal plans that will fit anyone's life, work, or play schedule.

Part III: Recipes

Whether you're a novice or pro in the kitchen, you'll appreciate these quick and easy recipes designed to boost your metabolic rate. By incorporating optimal food combinations and a variety of spices and flavors, you won't get bored or feel deprived and you'll keep your metabolism revved all day long. This part is separated into chapters containing recipes for breakfast, lunch, dinner, and snacks/desserts.

Part IV: Health and Lifestyle Issues

This part is focused on strategies to stick to healthy habits no matter what, whether you're traveling or at a party or dining out with your family. You'll find workouts you can do anytime, anywhere. You'll find out that activity doesn't have to mean spending hours at the gym. You'll learn how to build and sustain a powerful support system to help you stay on track. Also in this part, I address specific hormone-disrupting conditions you may face throughout your lifetime and provide specific recommendations for each.

Part V: The Part of Tens

A trademark of the *For Dummies* series, The Part of Tens gives you concise reference info to know about your metabolism. I give you sure-fire ways to know you've boosted your metabolic rate, dispel oh-so-common myths about metabolism, and suggest ten ways to beat those nagging cravings and unhealthy habits once and for all.

Icons Used in This Book

If you haven't gotten the hint already, books in the *For Dummies* series are designed to make information as accessible as possible for you to absorb and practice. I use icons throughout the book to help you identify the type of info you're about to read or give you a pass to skip it if you'd prefer.

This icon indicates that you're about to be enlightened with a nugget of wisdom that you can apply to your life to boost your metabolism.

This icon points out information to squirrel away in your mind and carry with you as you read this book. Some of them remind you *why* you're making these lifestyle changes, so that you stay motivated on your journey.

The icon flags stuff to watch out for and avoid, and identifies things that can prevent you from creating a safe and healthy environment for your lifestyle change.

You can skip the stuff next to this icon — it's not essential for your quest to boost your metabolism. But if you want more info on the scientific background, it's here for you to read.

Where to Go from Here

Well, now it's time you get started. Try reading the first chapter for a basic foundation of what you'll get with a boosted metabolism so that you're motivated to start your journey. But if you have ADD or simply want more specific info on what to eat with sample meal plans, skip to Part II. If you want to cook something great for your metabolism tonight, go directly to Part III, and if you feel like working out, head to Chapter 11. My hope is that, no matter where you start, you'll take away information that will help you on a path to better health and a maximized metabolism.

Don't feel overwhelmed! Taking small steps for change is better in the long run than a complete (likely unrealistic) overhaul of your habits. Be patient. Remember that your happy and healthy life is dictated by much more than a number on the scale. Take this book tip by tip, chapter by chapter, until you're at a place where you wake up and you know you're doing the best you can for your metabolism.

Part I

Getting Started with Boosting Your Metabolism

In this part . . .

- ✔ Discover what metabolism is and how your metabolic rate affects your weight and your life.
- ✔ Understand how metabolism governs the storage and burning of calories.
- ✔ Get the real dirt on restrictive diets and find out how achieving balance in your eating habits works in the long term.
- ✔ Figure out what speeds up and slows down your metabolism.
- ✔ Calculate your nutritional needs to boost your metabolism.

Chapter 1

Metabolism 101: Understanding How It Works

· ·

In This Chapter

▶ Defining metabolism and calories and understanding their role in your health and life

▶ Balancing energy storage and use

▶ Recognizing the roles of nutrients and hormones

▶ Understanding how deprivation diets are bad for your metabolism and weight

· ·

You've probably heard the word *metabolism* being thrown around with the latest fad diet craze, in nutrition and fitness articles, on talk shows, and from gym rats. They all claim to know the best way to boost your metabolism so that you can lose a lot of weight in a little time. You may actually believe many misconceptions about metabolism and weight. By the end of this book, you'll know better.

If it weren't for your metabolism, you wouldn't be alive. Your metabolism isn't just a vehicle to blame for your weight-loss woes. It's a machine that impacts your energy and stress levels, your sleeping habits, and your long-term health. Every cell in your body is involved in a process associated with your metabolic rate.

Unfortunately, instead of health, *thinness* has become idealized in the United States, and extreme dieting and weight-loss methods are used to achieve that ideal. Because of our nation's obesity epidemic, this dichotomy causes nutrition messages to get all jumbled in the media and likely your social circle, and you may come to believe these mixed messages as truth. So, congratulations on taking the first step and picking up this book. Clearly you want the truth about what metabolism is and how it really affects your weight!

This chapter breaks down metabolism step by step so that, by the end of it, you'll understand why many of the "truths" you've believed are actually doing you more harm than good.

Introducing Metabolism

It's time for you to meet your metabolism and become friends. Because being enemies with your metabolism, blaming it for your weight struggles, and fighting it in an effort to reach your goals aren't going to get you anywhere. Instead, once you learn the basics about how your metabolism operates, you're able to work together with yours, to maximize your metabolic rate and get to where you want to be with your weight and health.

Metabolism is life

On the most basic level, *metabolism* is the process by which your body converts the food and water you consume into energy for immediate use or to be stored for later. This energy doesn't only power your jog — every action your body performs, including brushing your teeth and getting dressed in the morning, requires this energy.

Your muscles aren't the only organs that need to be fueled. Your lungs, heart, and brain all require the energy generated in your metabolism powerhouse. But when you eat *more* than your body needs for all its functions, your metabolism stores that energy as (drumroll, please) ... fat.

Your metabolism is never sleeping or completely broken; its processes are going on every minute of every day. Of course, your metabolism may not be maximized to work the best it can — but that's what you're here to fix.

Everyone has to eat and drink, but your body could go for weeks without food. Your metabolism is programmed to conserve the energy for when you absolutely need it. In the absence of food, your metabolism actually slow down and releases less energy at a time so that you can survive longer.

But without water, you'd be dead within a few days. That's because:

- ✔ Your body is more than 60 percent water.

- ✔ The cells in your body that make up your skin, heart, lungs, and muscles (and everything else) require water to maintain their size and shape.

- ✔ Water helps regulate your body temperature. In the process of creating energy from the food you eat, your metabolism generates heat. You sweat when you're overheated to release that heat from your body, and you drink water to replenish the water loss.

- ✔ Compounds involved in metabolic reactions that help your body process and create energy require water to operate.

The Kreb's cycle

In high school biology, you learned about the Kreb's, or citric acid, cycle. This is the chemical reaction that's at the heart of generating energy, or heat, from breaking down *macronutrients* — carbohydrates, protein, and fats — into metabolites to create energy your body can use.

✔ All *aerobic* organisms (ones that breathe air) undergo these step-by-step reactions to break down food into energy.

✔ In the absence of oxygen, for example during anaerobic exercise, which is short-lived, high-intensity movement, the cycle still occurs, but less energy is created, requiring your body to "make up for it" afterwards (see Chapter 11).

✔ *Mitochondria* are the units in your cells where the reactions occur. They're also known as "cellular power plants."

✔ The Kreb's cycle requires two molecules of H_2O (water).

✔ Vitamins, particularly the B vitamins, and minerals such as calcium and magnesium play a big role in facilitating each step.

✔ *Enzymes* are proteins with an *–ase* at the end of their name (such as dehydrogenase) that are catalysts for the reactions.

✔ The cycle produces adenosine triphosphate, or ATP, which is released to do work wherever it's needed, for example, repairing muscle tissue after weight-bearing exercise. To function, your body burns ATP like a car burns gasoline, which would make the Kreb's cycle kind of like an oil refinery.

Metabolism is at the foundation of your basic functioning to live. It's what makes your body smart in times of crisis, but it's also what hurts you if you're not eating enough or aren't eating the right types of foods. Later in this chapter, I talk more about restrictive diets and how they're harmful to your health.

Comprehending calories

You're either thinking about how many calories you burned through exercise or how many you need to cut, right? You're not thinking about what calories *are*. Whenever I explain calories, I always think back to the day I learned what a calorie truly is.

So what is it? A *calorie* is a measure of heat that's released from food when digested. More exactly, a calorie is the amount of heat needed to raise the temperature of 1 gram of water by 1 degree Celsius. 1,000 calories = 1 *kilocalorie*, or one Calorie — which is actually what *1 calorie* on a food label means. It's confusing, I know. What you have thought of as calories are actually kilocalories or Calories, but you can still call them calories because everyone else does, and I'll call them calories in this book from now on. Is that clear? Never mind. The more heat released, the more calories a food contains.

It wasn't until nutritional biochemistry lab in my junior year of college that all this really clicked for me, thanks to an experiment. We were each told to bring in a food item from a fast-food joint. I brought in a Big Mac from McDonald's. We ground it up and placed a portioned sample of the food in a *bomb calorimeter*, which has two chambers, one inside the other. The food is burned in the inside chamber, which is filled with oxygen, and in the outside chamber a certain amount of cold water is monitored for rises in temperature. The temperature increase correlated to about 500 calories for the whole Big Mac — which is what McDonald's had listed in the restaurant.

Of course, that lab example doesn't emulate exactly what's going on in your body when food is digested, but that's the gist of it.

You can also estimate how many calories are in a food if you know the protein, carbohydrate, and fat content.

- ✔ 1 gram of protein = 4 calories
- ✔ 1 gram of carbohydrate = 4 calories
- ✔ 1 gram of fat = 9 calories

For example, if you know that a certain amount of fat-free Greek yogurt contains 0 grams of fat, 7 grams of carbohydrate, and 18 grams of protein, you can expect that food to contain 100 calories.

There's also a discrepancy in calorie content among foods when they're cooked, raw, processed, or whole. A lot of that is due in part to the *thermic effect* of food (TEF), which accounts for the fact that some of the calories you eat are burned off during the digestion process itself. Therefore, the net amount of calories that make it into your body's energy system is actually less than what's initially present in the food. An interesting study published in *Food and Nutrition Research* studied two groups of people. One group ate multigrain bread with cheddar cheese, and another ate white bread with processed cheese — both containing the same proportion of calories from fat, carbohydrate, and protein. The study found the following:

- ✔ Whole foods have a larger thermic effect (use up more energy to break down) than processed foods do and therefore have fewer calories left over to potentially get stored as fat.

- ✔ There was no difference in satiation (feeling of fullness) reported, yet the average energy expended with the processed cheese sandwich was 50 percent less than the whole-foods sandwich!

✔ The moral of the story here is that, although technically you consume fewer calories from the whole-food sandwich, you feel as satisfied as you would from the processed sandwich.

Unfortunately, in the U.S., we eat about 30 percent more processed foods — such as frozen dinners and pre-made meals — than we do fresh, whole foods. These convenience foods, expanding portion sizes, and more sedentary lifestyles all contribute to the growing obesity epidemic that affects about a third of Americans.

Foods with a higher TEF help improve your metabolic rate. Fat is relatively easy to break down and therefore has a low TEF, whereas protein and complex carbohydrates are more difficult to digest and so have a higher TEF. And of course, fiber, the complex carbohydrate found in many whole grains, fruits, and vegetables, is mostly indigestible to begin with! The bottom line is that *whole foods that contain lean protein and fiber help keep you fuller, longer, and can help you lose weight.* (You'll find more on the thermic effect of food and how it impacts your metabolic rate in Chapter 3.)

Balancing using energy and storing it

Metabolism is a two-step process between catabolism and anabolism. The balance between the two is controlled by *hormones,* chemicals released by cells that have specific functions. Hormones are either classified as anabolic or catabolic depending on what they do:

✔ **Catabolism** breaks down macronutrients into their smaller units to release energy for physical activity or to use for anabolism. For example, the catabolic hormone cortisol is released in response to stress, causing your body to break down muscle protein to use for energy.

✔ **Anabolism** builds up larger molecules from smaller units requiring units of energy — for example, creating hormones, enzymes, and compounds for cell growth to build bone and muscles. The anabolic hormone insulin, for example, controls the amount of glucose in your blood by converting it into compounds that cells can use or store. The sex hormones testosterone and estrogen are also anabolic hormones that work to develop male and female sex characteristics.

Your body weight depends on your body's catabolism minus anabolism, or the amount of energy your body takes up to use. If your catabolism greatly exceeds anabolism, the excess energy generated is stored as glycogen (for later use by your muscles) or fat (which serves to increase body weight). Many factors impact which state your body favors, and everyone is different.

Here are some reasons your metabolism may be on the fritz:

- **Calorie intake:** If you're eating more calories than you can use, your body will store them for later. See Chapter 3 to calculate how many calories your body needs to function on a baseline level and with added activity.

- **Activity level:** If you're not active enough, aren't doing any weight-resistant exercise to work your muscles, or are too active that your body is stressed, you can be said to be in a more *catabolic state*.

- **Age:** One reason why losing weight becomes more difficult as you age is that levels of your anabolic hormones which use up that excess energy, like testosterone or estrogen, decrease, resulting in decreased muscle mass and increased fat storage.

- **Genetics and hormone-disrupting conditions:** Based on individual differences in genetics, you may be more or less prone to a sluggish metabolism. Also hormone-disrupting conditions like menopause and hypothyroid play a role (read more about this in Chapter 12).

For more on the factors that impact your metabolic rate, see Chapter 2.

Weighing benefits beyond weight loss

Although boosting your metabolism helps your body burn and use up more calories so you can lose weight, it also works to improve your health. (But your weight doesn't tell you everything about your health status. Some people are underweight with a sluggish metabolism, and some are overweight with a faster one.)

If you choose less processed foods and more wholesome nutrients, don't go too many hours between meals, and make a commitment to regular activity, you'll benefit from a range of positive side effects, in addition to weight loss, including the following:

- More energy
- Better sleep
- Improved mood and concentration
- Stronger immune system
- Stronger muscles and better mobility
- Improved blood glucose control with diabetes
- Improved blood pressure and heart health

Something to digest

Digestion actually begins with the enzymes in your saliva starting to break down nutrients in your mouth. Foods that take longer to digest typically help boost your metabolism because the more work your body does, the more heat or calories it requires your body to use.

✔ **Mouth:** Chewing breaks down the food, and the enzyme amylase, in your saliva, begins breaking down starch into simple sugars.

✔ **Stomach:** The enzyme pepsin in your stomach starts breaking down proteins, and other factors work on carbohydrates and fats as well.

✔ **Small intestine:** This is where most of the digestion and absorption takes place. The small intestine contains small fingerlike structures called villi that absorb nutrients into your bloodstream once they're broken into their simplest form. These nutrients first get processed by the liver to filter out anything harmful, like alcohol and toxins. Then the good parts get passed along to your cells for energy. What the small intestine can't absorb, like fiber, water, and bacteria, gets transferred to the large intestine.

✔ **Large intestine:** This is your body's last-ditch effort to absorb any nutrients, and the rest gets passed out of your body.

Meeting the Macronutrients

The nutrients you consume in the largest amounts — carbohydrates, protein, and fat — are known as macronutrients. You require all three to provide you with the energy you need and optimize your metabolic rate. A restrictive diet which focuses on cutting out one of them — fat or carbohydrates, for example — can cause fatigue, increased food cravings, and lead to other vitamin or mineral deficiencies.

You also need vitamins and minerals but in smaller amounts, so they're called *micronutrients*. Also, you do require water in large amounts, but it's not technically a food or nutrient.

This section reviews each of the three macronutrients, why you need 'em, and how they fit into the metabolism puzzle.

Facts about fat

Of all the macronutrients, the most confusion surrounds fat and cholesterol. You may automatically think, "If I eat fat, I'll get fat." It's true that the American diet is a rich source of fat, and too much fat can have negative health impacts such as increased cholesterol, heart disease, and weight gain. However, although fat is a concentrated source of calories, and too much can be bad for you, you still need to eat fat for essential functions:

- ✔ It's a readily available source of energy for use in metabolism (the highest concentration of energy at 9 calories per gram).
- ✔ It supplies fatty acids for use in developing hormones such as your sex and hunger hormones.
- ✔ It's required for the absorption of fat-soluble vitamins A, D, E, and K.
- ✔ It helps satisfy you by improving taste and variety in meals so that you aren't hungry again soon after.
- ✔ Even when fat is stored, it helps keep your body temperature regulated and protects organs from damage.

Anything you eat in excess of what your body can use for energy gets stored as fat, not just the fat you eat. To reduce your body fat, focus on a balanced diet in which you get about 20–35 percent of your calories from fat, to keep your metabolic rate up and so that you don't feel deprived. This doesn't mean that 30 percent of what you eat can come from fat. Each fat gram contains 9 calories so you need to consume about half the amount of fat grams that you would from carbohydrates or protein for the same calories. For example:

- ✔ 1 ounce of pistachios = 7 grams of fat, 80 calories
- ✔ 1 ounce (1 slice) of whole wheat bread = 15 grams of carbohydrate, 80 calories

Most fats in food, no matter the type, are in the form of triglycerides. *Triglycerides* are composed of three fatty acid molecules connected by a compound known as *glycerol*. When the body needs fat for energy, the triglyceride is broken down by the enzyme lipase through lipolysis into the free fatty acids, which can then enter the Kreb's cycle to generate energy and transport oxygen through the blood.

- ✔ During high-intensity exercise, although carbohydrates are the main source of fuel, fats are needed to access glycogen, which is the stored form of carbohydrates.
- ✔ Fat is the main fuel source for low-intensity exercise for longer periods of time.

For more on how your body uses fuel during exercise, see Chapter 11.

Not all fats are created equal when it comes to your health. Table 1-1 outlines each type of fat from good to bad and where to find them.

Table 1-1	Facts About Fat Types	
Type	**Description**	**Sources**
Unsaturated	Lower risk of heart disease. Omega-3s have additional benefits and increase hormones to signal satiety (see Chapter 5 for more)	Olive oil, fish, nuts, avocado, soybeans
Saturated	Linked to heart disease and high cholesterol (see Chapter 4 for more)	Meat, butter, milk, cheese, egg yolks
Trans	Man-made fat which increases cholesterol and impacts glucose breakdown, slowing metabolism	Commercially packaged baked goods and breads, frozen foods, condiments

Although boosting your metabolism means getting rid of unwanted body fat, you still need *some* stored fat for essential functions such as providing energy and absorbing the fat-soluble vitamins A, D, E, K. See Chapter 3 for how much fat to eat and how to measure your progress through measuring body fat percentage.

Clarifying carbohydrates

Ever since Dr. Atkins came out with his carbohydrate-hating, protein-loving diet, you've seen more and more products hit the shelves with low-carb claims and more people banishing bagels and pasta from their diets. But carbohydrates truly are our main fuel source for metabolism and provide energy to our muscles and brain cells.

There was a shift in the types of carbs Americans consume as we went from a rural society to a more industrialized one: we're eating more processed sugars and sweeteners than ever before. This is what's attributed to an increase in obesity and health conditions — not carbohydrates from wholesome, natural sources like whole grains, fruits, and vegetables.

Carbohydrates are in food as simple carbohydrates and complex carbohydrates.

Simple carbohydrates include the following:

- ✔ **Monosaccharides** are the simplest form of carb and contain only one sugar molecule. Examples include glucose, fructose, and galactose.
- ✔ **Disaccharides** contain two sugar molecules linked together. Examples: lactose, maltose, and sucrose.

Complex carbohydrates include starch and fiber, which are simple sugars strung together by the hundreds or thousands.

Fiber isn't broken down the same way as the other carbohydrates. Depending on whether the fiber is soluble or insoluble, it's either broken down into a gel form (soluble) or not really digested at all. Fiber helps keep you fuller longer than any carbohydrate-containing food and is a major metabolism booster. Find out why in Chapter 5.

Besides fiber, no matter where your carbohydrate comes from, it's broken down into glucose to either get utilized for energy or stored for later as fat. It takes longer to break down the chains in complex carbohydrates for use as energy, which is why they make you feel fuller longer, without the rapid highs and lows in your blood glucose levels like you get with simple sugars.

The body uses glucose as part of metabolism in many ways:

- ✔ Glucose is used immediately in the Kreb's cycle to create energy.
- ✔ Glucose is converted into glycogen by the liver and muscles to supply energy when needed.
- ✔ When the muscle and liver stores are full, your liver turns the excess glucose into fat stores. When needed, those can be burned for fuel, but can't be converted back to glucose.

Your brain requires glucose to think, remember, and act. Therefore, restricting carbohydrates too much can be detrimental to your metabolism because your judgment is lowered, you feel deprived, and you'll be more likely to overeat later on. Just as with fats and proteins, choosing the right kinds of carbohydrates is key to achieving that balance between storing and using energy the best you can. Chapter 5 talks more about the best kinds of carbs to boost your metabolic rate.

Picturing protein

Protein is the second-most prominent feature in your body after water. The brain, muscles, skin, blood, hair, and nails are all comprised of *amino acids*, the building blocks that make up protein. The antibodies that fight infection, as well as enzymes, which are the catalysts for lots of the metabolism reactions, are built from protein too.

So, protein on its own isn't a readily available source of energy for your body, but you need protein to help process the other two macronutrients, fat and carbohydrate, for energy. In addition, a small amount of protein also serves to create hormones like insulin, which regulates the amount of glucose in your blood.

 When it comes to your metabolism, building and maintaining lean muscle mass is protein's primary goal. Muscle mass burns more calories at rest than fat mass does and is therefore very precious to any metabolism-conscious person. There's a lot of protein turnover, and your body needs to constantly supply the tissues with amino acids as they get broken down to be built up again.

When you do resistance exercises like using weights, the tissue in your muscles gets broken down and needs to be repaired with a new influx of amino acids coming from the protein you eat in your diet.

 Every food contains protein except for pure oil, but the composition of amino acids varies. Some foods offer up a better combo than others:

- ✔ *High-quality* proteins are ones that contain all the essential nine amino acids you need to eat (because your body can't make them). These are mainly proteins from animals: meat, dairy, and eggs.

- ✔ *Low-quality* proteins, or incomplete proteins, are from vegetable sources like beans, grains, and vegetables. However, by combining two vegetarian foods together, you can retrieve all the amino acids your body needs. Examples include pairing rice and beans, tofu with rice and vegetables, or peanut butter on whole-wheat bread.

Experts used to think that because the body doesn't store amino acids, as it stores fats and carbs, you'd have to pair low-quality proteins at the same meal. Although that may still be true for children, it's not so important for adults. As long as you have complementary proteins throughout the day, you'll meet your needs.

The bottom line is that your body is resourceful, and when you have too much or too little of any of the macronutrients — fat, carbohydrate, or protein — there are consequences for your metabolism. Table 1-2 shows why having a balance of all three helps boost your metabolism and keeps your body working the best it can.

Table 1-2	Macronutrient Under/Over Effects	
Macronutrient	*Not Enough*	*Too Much*
Fat	Vitamin deficiencies	Stored as fat
Carbohydrate	Low energy, impaired digestion, dehydration	Stress on pancreas to produce insulin, stored as fat
Protein	Lose lean muscle	In absence of carbohydrate, fat is processed for energy, which puts stress on your kidneys

Recognizing the Role of Hormones

Once the food you eat gets broken down, that's when hormones jump into action. They not only help monitor what's absorbed but also how those nutrients are used by your body. Hormones communicate messages from one cell to another, and certain cells are programmed to understand the messages of only specific hormones. In this section, I outline the four main need-to-know hormones and their role in your metabolism.

Basically, *hormones* are chemicals which are released from your endocrine glands into your bloodstream to be used by your body. (Your *exocrine* glands, sweat and salivary glands, release secretions onto the outside of your body.)

The endocrine glands, such as the thyroids and adrenals as well as other organs like your kidneys, produce and release hormones. These chemicals are at the center of your metabolism, making sure your body is operating the way it should to either burn or store energy and impacting how effectively you're able to lose weight.

Your metabolism may be sluggish because these hormones are affected by your diet, lifestyle, and even your genes. Chapter 12 reviews a few hormone-disrupting conditions like diabetes, menopause, and thyroid disease which cause many metabolism woes.

You can make changes to your diet to help get your hormones working for you and boost your metabolic rate.

Glucose has an "in" with insulin

Insulin, a hormone produced by the beta cells of your pancreas, regulates carbohydrate and fat metabolism:

- ✔ It's released when it senses carbohydrate or protein in your blood as they're being digested.
- ✔ It causes your cells to take up glucose to be used for energy or to store either in the liver or muscle as glycogen or in your fat cells as triglycerides.
- ✔ When present, insulin stops your body from breaking down stored fat to use for energy.
- ✔ Insulin stimulates protein synthesis and encourages amino acid uptake by your muscles.

When your metabolism is working at its peak, your body has feedback mechanisms to regulate the amount of insulin your body makes so there's neither too much nor too little. That way, you're using glucose appropriately for energy and not storing too much fat.

If you have diabetes, your body either doesn't make enough (or any!) insulin or your body doesn't respond well to it, which is known as *insulin resistance*. But if your cells aren't as receptive to insulin, there are ways to help reverse that. By seeking out medical care, making changes to your diet and activity levels, and achieving a healthy weight, you can regulate your blood glucose.

"Stress"-ing cortisol

Cortisol is produced by your adrenal glands and is released in response to stress. It has many primary functions in the metabolism realm and basically functions to make energy available if needed for quick use, like if you need to escape from a risky situation (also known as the fight or flight response) or even to face a challenging day at the office. Cortisol is within a class of hormones called *glucocorticoid* and it increases blood glucose levels:

- ✔ It works against insulin to keep glucose around and breaks down glucose from stored fat to release energy (through a process called gluconeogenesis).

✔ It reduces protein uptake (those proteins are used in gluconeogenesis) by the muscles. So, if cortisol is around for long periods of time, it can lead to a reduction in lean muscle mass.

✔ The release of cortisol increases blood pressure.

✔ Cortisol suppresses the immune system because those functions aren't vital to surviving an immediate threat or stressful situation.

The problem is that over time, our stressful situations don't necessarily require an energy release. If you're sedentary at your job and are experiencing stress, you aren't using up that circulating glucose that cortisol makes available for you. Therefore, that excess can get re-stored as fat, particularly abdominal fat.

In my online article "Taking Care to Change Your Lifestyle", you can read more on how your lifestyle affects your cortisol levels, metabolism, and the steps you can start taking today for change. Briefly, the factors in your life that may be causing an increase in cortisol include the following:

✔ You're not sleeping enough or getting at least seven hours of sleep per night.

✔ You're not active enough. Regular exercise helps reduces anxiety.

✔ You're drinking too much caffeine. Stick to one cup per day or less to minimize the rise in cortisol.

✔ You don't have a balanced diet or are lacking B vitamins and magnesium, which help lower cortisol and boost your immune system.

The thyroid connection

The thyroid is an endocrine gland in your neck that's responsible for regulating the pace at which your metabolism is working. It basically uses the iodine you consume in foods to produce two main hormones called T3 and T4. Every single cell in your body responds to these hormones to either pick up the pace or slow down when it comes to converting oxygen and calories to energy. More specifically, your thyroid hormones:

✔ Encourage normal growth and development in your whole body.

✔ Speed up all of insulin's activities.

✔ Enhance the body's response to stress hormones.

✔ Regulate your body temperature.

The most common cause of any abnormality with your thyroid is due to a genetic autoimmune disease where your body attacks its own cells. If your thyroid is working too slowly, your body isn't able to transfer calories to energy, and they may be more easily stored as fat. That's why people with hypothyroid may gain weight or have difficulty losing weight. With hypothyroid, your ability to build up or break down proteins, fats, and carbohydrates is slowed — and that ability is at the core of your metabolic rate.

But all hope isn't lost with a thyroid diagnosis. By following the metabolism-boosting plan in this book, you can still lose weight at a steady rate. For more tips specific to the thyroid diet, check out Chapter 12.

Hungry for hunger hormones

If you've lost weight, only to gain it back, you may be all too familiar with your hunger and satiety hormones. *Leptin* and *ghrelin* are your body's main hormones that regulate when you're hungry and when you're full and may be the key to your metabolism and body weight.

Leptin is what makes you feel full:

- ✔ It's secreted by fat cells, and the more fat you have, the more leptin is secreted.

- ✔ Leptin signals to the thyroid that there's adequate fat so you burn it off instead of keep storing it up. The problem that comes into play with obesity is that you can develop resistance to leptin over time.

- ✔ Your body may think you're starving because of leptin resistance, or because you're not eating adequately (such as when you're on a too restrictive diet). So, what happens, then?

- ✔ You increase fat storage instead of burning and burn less calories overall.

- ✔ Your appetite increases, you don't feel satisfied, and you're more likely to overeat.

- ✔ You're more likely to develop insulin resistance.

If you've been overweight for awhile, it's harder for you to lose weight. But it's definitely not impossible. This is where activity plays a major role in helping to burn off more calories and stabilize your hormones. Chapter 11 highlights metabolism-boosting moves to help jump-start weight loss.

Ghrelin is the hormone I call the "hunger gremlin," because it's the one that increases your appetite:

- It's made in your stomach and tells your brain to eat or drink when your stomach is empty.

- It also controls genes that hold on to fats instead of burning them off.

- Research shows that when you're sleep deprived, your ghrelin levels are elevated, and leptin levels are depressed, which is why you're hungrier after a few sleepless nights.

- Studies also suggest that when you skip breakfast, high-calorie foods are more appealing to you due to the ghrelin's powers.

Your response to these hunger hormones may differ from the person standing next to you. Just as everyone's metabolism is different, the way a body copes with stress and hormones and nutrients isn't the same for everyone. Your environment, diet, and lifestyle can affect how your metabolism reacts, and that's what this book addresses. On some level, metabolism can be a mystery, but you can take actionable steps to change the hand you've been dealt.

Let's talk about sex hormones

Whether you're a man or woman, the hormones testosterone and estrogen play a leading role in your metabolism. Most notably, your sex hormones impact your body composition, which may be seen with a glance at the male and female physiques. Males tend to have more muscle mass and burn more calories at rest, which is why men can typically eat more and not gain weight. For women, it may seem like whatever you eat goes straight to your thighs and hips, and it's more difficult to lose fat.

Estrogen

Estrogen is the hormone that's integral for reproduction as well as development of sex characteristics like breast tissue. The hormone, which is produced in your ovaries, adrenal glands, and fat tissue also protects cognitive functioning, promotes healthy bones, and helps control your cholesterol levels.

During menopause, estrogen levels rapidly decline, resulting in the following:

- **Increased conversion of calories to fat:** Because fat cells also make estrogen, your body favors being in fat storage mode to increase those cells and promote estrogen production.

✔ **Hot flashes that can interrupt your sleep:** Not getting a good night's sleep contributes to alterations in your hunger hormones with negative metabolism effect.

✔ **Mood swings that can impact what you eat:** You may crave more fatty foods or sweets.

See Chapter 12 for more info on menopause and how diet and exercise can help balance you out and boost your metabolic rate.

Testosterone

Testosterone, on the other hand, is produced by both males and females but is more prominent in males. It's produced primarily in the testes in men, and in the ovaries in women. Testosterone

✔ Promotes protein synthesis and increases muscle mass function.

✔ Promotes endurance, which helps with activity and exercise.

✔ Helps prevent heart disease by keeping cholesterol and triglyceride levels in check.

Human growth hormone: Fountain of youth?

Human Growth Hormone (also known as HGH) is a hormone produced by the pituitary gland in your brain and is released during childhood and adolescence. Production of this hormone starts decreasing steadily in your 20s. It's the hormone responsible for the part of metabolism. HGH

✔ Spurs growth and development of cell tissue and bones

✔ Promotes more muscle mass

✔ Decreases glucose storage so you use that for energy, shrinking fat cells

✔ Increases blood vessels and collagen, resulting in younger-looking skin

Synthetic production of HGH began in the 1950s to treat children who were not making enough of it due to an inborn genetic error. But now it's being used illegally in sports to increase muscle mass (it's one of the drugs that Lance Armstrong was accused of taking, which stripped him of his Tour de France titles). It is also prescribed under the table to women who want to look younger and lose weight.

Unfortunately, although HGH increases muscle mass, it's not proven to improve strength. And synthetic HGH has potential side effects, including insulin resistance, increased diabetes risk, and perhaps even promotion of cancer growth. The truth may be that synthetic HGH "cheats" Mother Nature and could shorten your life.

You can't alter HGH production with diet. In adulthood, it's released more during sleep. Just another reason why getting seven hours per night can boost your metabolism.

As with estrogen, your testosterone levels decrease after age 40, resulting in less muscle mass, more fat mass, and a more sluggish metabolic rate. Stress hormones also interfere with both estrogen and testosterone, reducing their metabolism-boosting effects even further at any age. As you age, losing weight becomes more and more difficult in large part because of these sex hormones. But through diet and exercise, you can work to balance out your hormones so that they're working for you rather than against you.

Why Other Diets Used to Work and Don't Now

In the past, you may have reached your goal weight just in time for your high school reunion. But then the holiday season came around and threw you off track, or you injured yourself and weren't able to go to the gym, or your life simply became too hectic and you ended up gaining all your weight back (or more).

Sound familiar? You may have also heard the terms *yo-yo dieting* and *yo-yo weight* because the truth is that losing and gaining is so common it's become part of American culture.

Everywhere you turn you see advertising for a diet plan with celebrity endorsements. "If she can look that way, so can I." Although these diets do have a goal to make you slim, often they're not concerned about your health. Being on too restrictive a diet hinders your healthy relationship with food. It may work in the short term, but it backfires later, setting you up for a weight rollercoaster the rest of your life.

You're reading this book because you want to make changes that last a lifetime, right? Not a quick fix (which doesn't exist). The metabolism-boosting plan in this book is meant to help you get there in ways that are realistic for you, one step at a time.

Your body on a diet

Believe me, I know how tempting it is to pick up a book that promises you'll lose 20 pounds in two weeks. You're bombarded with transformations of bodies on infomercials for the latest diet trends.

These changes aren't forever. They're quick fixes that can actually harm your health *and* your ability to lose weight, boost your metabolism, and live a long, healthy, happy life.

The dangers of the HCG diet

A diet that restricts calories and injects you with hormones to help you lose weight — sounds like the perfect combo? Think again. HCG, or Human Chorionic Gonadotropin, is a hormone normally produced during pregnancy. It's been approved by the FDA to treat infertility, but is illegal when sold for weight-loss purposes.

The HCG diet combines a mere *500 calories* per day from foods like organic meats, veggies, and fish (don't even think about eating any dairy, carbs, or alcohol) with shots of the hormone. If dieters have a slip, they're supposed to eat nothing but apples and water for 24 hours. The hormone supposedly helps stave off hunger and blasts fat. However the quick weight loss that may result is extremely harmful to your metabolism. It can cause severe muscle wasting, bone loss, as well as electrolyte imbalances — and can even be fatal. Not to mention, you can only keep this restriction up for so long, and then you'll go back to your old habits. Once you do, because your metabolism is out of whack, you'll not only gain the weight back very easily, but more often than not, you'll gain even more weight because your body is storing up on fat, unsure when you'll decide to deprive it again.

A *diet* is the quantity and quality of the foods you eat in your everyday life. Over the past few decades, the word *diet* has become synonymous with a restrictive weight-loss plan that inevitably cuts out your favorite foods or demonizes an entire food group like fat or carbohydrate.

There are a few intrinsic problems with the new definition of diet:

✔ When you cut out food groups, a slew of negative side effects can occur (covered earlier in this chapter).

✔ When you cut out the foods you love completely, you're *more* likely to crave and overeat those foods later.

✔ You develop an unhealthy relationship with food. Instead of thinking of food as fuel, it becomes just a means to gain or lose weight. You obsess and constantly think about what you're eating, social situations around food provoke anxiety, and you let food take over your life.

✔ On a physiological level, your body chemistry is altered when you restrict calories.

As you lose weight, your caloric needs also decrease. If you're 200 pounds, you need to eat about 1600 calories a day to lose weight. But at 150 pounds, your needs are closer to 1400 calories per day to continue losing weight at a steady rate. The less you weigh, the less you'll be burning at rest. Part of the reason is that your muscle fiber twitch is altered so that your muscles are actually burning off fewer calories than someone else who has been at 150 pounds forever.

Instead of turning to a drastic restrictive diet, when you're at a halt with your weight loss, it may just be time to reduce your calorie intake in your diet or increase the amount you burn with activity. In Chapter 3, you can estimate your metabolic rate, or *caloric burn*, and also learn about the more sophisticated methods of gaining a better understanding of the amount of calories you need to eat to lose weight.

Riding a weight rollercoaster

Once you hit your goal weight, it's smooth sailing, right? Not so much. Maintaining your weight is often even harder than losing weight in the first place:

- ✔ You've been depriving your body too much in ways that aren't realistic for you to sustain.

- ✔ Your hunger hormone ghrelin is elevated after a restrictive diet. Research also shows your brain is programmed to respond even more emotionally to decadent food cues after such a diet. Researchers found that the pleasure centers of your brain light up more when faced with fatty or sugary foods post-dieting. So, you may not be able to resist food like you could in the past.

- ✔ All your body's hormones are used to being overweight, so it almost actively fights to get back to the weight you were at before. That's why more gradual, slow weight loss is more likely to last long term, because you're giving your hormones time to adjust to the change in body weight.

It's hard to know how long the post-restrictive-diet vulnerable state persists, but experts think it could be for years. That doesn't mean it's impossible to maintain your weight, it's just much harder. Acknowledging that is the first step toward tackling the changes you can make. A huge part of stepping off of the weight rollercoaster ride is changing your thought process surrounding the foods you eat.

It's time to break those bad habits

It's hard to know which habits are genetic and which are due to your environment, but both play a role in your metabolic rate. You may have grown up in a household where everyone was a member of the Clean Plate Club, and your parents, or siblings were perpetually "on a diet." Studies suggest that some people are programmed in their genes to crave high-calorie foods. But you're also surrounded by fast-food joints, and with most social situations revolving around food, it becomes more difficult to avoid those foods and reprogram yourself psychologically.

It's easier said than done to reverse your mentality. But the more you focus on how you look and feel, and not just the number on the scale, the more you'll realize the long-term benefits of maximizing your metabolism the healthy way.

My goal is that you'll know the following when you finish this book:

- ✔ How to set realistic goals, both for the short term and long term
- ✔ How to challenge your thoughts about dieting and what a healthy lifestyle means
- ✔ The practical steps you can take to set yourself up for success with your new mentality
- ✔ How to take action with manageable changes to your diet and activity levels to maximize your metabolism for the long term!

Chapter 2

Your Metabolism and Your Daily Life

• •

In This Chapter

▶ Understanding what impacts your metabolism

▶ Diagnosing a sluggish metabolism

▶ Enjoying the lifelong benefits of boosting your metabolism

• •

*E*very day you make thousands of decisions about what to put into your body, which activities to engage in, and how you act. The outcome of these choices can affect your metabolism day in, day out. Although it's true that everyone is born into a unique body, I'm sorry to tell you that you can't simply place all the blame on your genes when it comes to your weight and health.

Living with a sluggish metabolism can literally be a drag. Not just a drag on your efforts to lose weight but also on your energy level, mood, appearance, physical health, and overall well-being. Using these markers, in addition to the number on the scale, will help keep you motivated for change. As you start to make healthier lifestyle choices, you can eliminate the symptoms of a sluggish metabolism so that you look and feel your very best.

This chapter talks about many reasons why your metabolism may not be working efficiently, including what's in your DNA and the unhealthy habits you've picked up along the way. After understanding how these habits affect your health, you can then start taking realistic steps for change.

Your Metabolism and You

I know many people, both clients and friends, who have thrown their hands in the air and said, "I give up. I have a slow metabolism and I can't lose weight." Does this sound familiar to you? Often it's easier to place blame on something, especially when you're not even sure what makes that something tick.

This section explores the major factors of your life that affect your metabolism. Sure, a few of these factors are beyond your control. But many are well within the realm of possibility for change. Instead of throwing your hands up, you'll realize there are many steps you can take to give your metabolism a makeover and improve your health.

Don't know much biology?

The *cell* is the basic unit of life, and your body is made up of billions and billions of them. Metabolism is the rate at which those cells transform and use energy for fuel, growth, and development. As you age throughout life, your cells change, and therefore your metabolic rate changes based on various factors. You're born with a set of genes that dictates your sex, height, and underlying weight and body composition — proportion of fat and muscle — all of which affect your metabolic rate. As you age, your weight and body composition change, which means that through the years so does your metabolic rate.

I don't mean to be a downer by reviewing these scientific facts. However, getting a grip on the uncontrollable stuff like this can help you realize where you started out and what to work on when it comes to the lifestyle changes you *can* make.

Your biology doesn't have to be your destiny when it comes to metabolism.

Weighing muscle and fat

Your body composition has a big impact on your metabolic rate. Your body is composed of fat mass and fat-free mass. Fat-free mass includes your muscle, organs, bones, skin, and so on. The proportion between the two can vary from person to person based on DNA, sex, age, and fitness level. The takeaway here is that muscle mass is metabolically active tissue that burns more calories than fat mass. The exact amount of calories burned by muscle is under debate. However, the more lean muscle mass your body has, the more calories it burns, and therefore the more efficiently your metabolism works.

Muscle mass is denser than fat and can weigh up to three times more than the same volume of fat. My clients sometimes get frustrated when starting a workout program because they aren't losing weight. I often have to remind them that they are probably losing fat but building muscle tissue, which will burn more calories at rest, even when they're just sitting around watching TV. Once again: Health is much more than the number on the scale.

Weight loss doesn't always equal body fat loss. You can lose weight in the form of lean muscle mass if you're following a restrictive diet or not fueling yourself properly for the exercise you're doing. When you lose that desirable calorie-burning muscle mass, you're not only causing your metabolism to slow down even further, but you're setting yourself up for failure when it comes to weight maintenance.

Men have more muscle

Over the years, I've had many husband-and-wife clients come into my office together for weight loss, and 90 percent of the time, the male has more success than the female. Often he makes one change, such as cutting out soda or juice, or simply starting to exercise, and is able to lose weight. Meanwhile she struggles to do everything she can with her diet, activity, and lifestyle but her weight doesn't budge for weeks.

One reason is that once men hit puberty, they typically develop 20–40 percent more muscle mass than women, making their metabolic rates higher. Why is this so? Men produce more of the hormone testosterone, which promotes muscle development, and women are actually genetically engineered to have more body fat in preparation for pregnancy and lactation. On top of that, once women hit pre-menopause and menopause, their metabolism-boosting sex hormone, estrogen, drops, and a sluggish metabolism ensues. Typically, women gain about a pound or two per year during this time, and taking the weight off becomes more difficult. Chapter 12 talks more about menopause and how it affects your metabolism.

Losing muscle as you age

Do you remember when you could eat anything you wanted without putting on a pound? And now you gain weight just looking at a plate of French fries? The truth is that as you get older, your muscle mass declines. After age 20, your metabolic rate slows down between 5–10 percent each decade due to less lean muscle mass and more fat mass.

If you aren't doing any muscle-building activity, and you need 1,900 calories to maintain your weight at age 20, your calorie need could decrease to 1,750 calories at age 30, 1,650 at 40, 1,500 at 50, 1,350 at 60, and down to 1,300 by age 70. Over 50 years, that's 600 fewer calories that your body needs daily to maintain the same height and weight. Research also shows that it's not just body composition that changes as you age. Your organs, such as your heart and lungs, also seem to require fewer calories as you get older. At each decade milestone, you need to re-evaluate how you eat and how you move to stay within a healthy weight range.

How your height and weight relate

The bigger you are, the more calories you will burn at rest. Your body simply requires more calories for energy to fuel the larger mass. If you're taller, your metabolic rate is naturally higher. But if you're short, don't fret! A 2010 study in the *Journal of Experimental Biology* found that shorter people burn more calories when in motion — because they need to take more steps to cover the same distance when walking. That means that if your genes have dealt you a short stature, physical activity can make up the difference.

When you're overweight, you also need more calories due to more surface area of your body, and therefore your metabolism is actually faster. This is why it is often easier to lose weight when you have more to lose. As you begin to lose body mass, your caloric needs become less and less. This is one reason why healthy weight maintenance may be even more difficult than the process of losing the weight.

The genes you're wearing

If you have a friend who is the same sex, age, weight, and height, if you eat the same amount of calories and exercise together, it's possible one of you would gain weight and the other wouldn't. Your genes control not only your physical characteristics like height and weight, but also regulation of hormones, appetite signals, and risk for acquiring disease — all biochemical aspects that affect your metabolic rate. Because each person is born with a different set of DNA, each person has a unique metabolism, and some may use calories more efficiently than others. It doesn't seem fair, but even though you're taking in the same number of calories as your friend, she may be able to burn those calories for energy while you store them as fat.

Now for the good news! The way your genes act throughout your life is greatly affected by your environment. Factors like diet, exercise, and medication can actually turn the expression of certain genes on or off.

Nutrigenomics

Traditionally, most nutrition research was focused on nutrient deficiencies and how that affects health. *Nutrigenomics* is an emerging field that connects nutrient intake and gene expression. Nutrigenomics shows promise for personalized nutrition plans based on your unique DNA. More specifically, your risk for disease can be evaluated, and a certain "diet prescription" can be created to help reduce your risk. Although proper nutrition can mean disease prevention on its own, nutrigenomics may provide an early detection of sorts, with a more individualized solution.

It can be easy to get overwhelmed, but overhauling everything about your lifestyle all at once will likely not be realistic in the long term. Taking smaller steps to change one aspect at a time is a more manageable and sustainable way to reach your goals. As a bonus, it's easier.

You are what you eat

Have you ever stopped to think about what that really means? Metabolism is the foundation of life, and each of your cells requires nutrients to grow, develop, and maintain life within your body. So quite literally, your body is built upon not only what you eat, but how you consume food — how much you eat, when you eat, and what you drink.

The quality of your diet

Because metabolism involves breaking down proteins, fats, and carbohydrates for fuel, the higher quality of that fuel, the more efficiently your body can use it. Food is like gas for your car — you can't just put anything in your tank. High-quality lean proteins, heart-healthy fatty acids, and high-fiber carbohydrates are the types of macronutrients (the nutrients you need the largest doses of in your diet) that give your body the best mileage when it comes to metabolism and energy. In addition, certain vitamins and minerals in your diet make sure your body functions as best it can. In Chapter 5, I review these nutrients and how to include them in your diet.

Whole foods — ones which are unprocessed or unrefined — contain more nutrients at-the-ready to fuel the cells of your body and keep your metabolism efficiently burning those calories. Throughout this book, you will discover the best foods for your metabolism and how to incorporate them into your diet on a daily basis. You will also find out which processed foods to avoid and which aren't so bad.

There is no single villain in your diet that causes weight gain. It's important to look at the big picture.

Identifying your eating behaviors

Too often people focus only on the types of food they're eating and not enough on their behaviors surrounding food and drink. You may have read and heard a lot about *what* to eat, but *how* you eat is very important for metabolism. Do you fall into one of the following eating behavior categories?

Overeating

Hormones regulate your appetite and the signals to your brain that tell you when you're hungry and when you're stuffed. Research shows that when people overeat for many weeks, those signals may be disrupted. It can be a double whammy — not only is your metabolism slower, but you're more likely to continue overeating. Your body will convert any calories that it doesn't need into fat, which can cause weight gain and increased risk for disease down the road.

Undereating

Undereating also can slow your metabolism — by up to 20 percent. It's a survival mechanism. Your body thinks its being deprived, and instead of burning calories it holds on to them and stores them as fat for later use. Your body will literally slow down its functions because it doesn't have the proper calories to keep it moving, just as your car may peter out when low on gas. In addition, if you're not eating enough, you're likely losing that precious muscle mass, not fat mass. Again, your body is very smart, and in case you're in an emergency situation this process allows you to survive longer without food. But for someone trying to lose weight, this is obviously not an effective strategy.

That's why it's so important to know what your body needs and how to fuel it with the proper balance of nutrients. By blindly following a fad or restrictive diet, or by over-exercising, you may lose weight in the short term, but you can slow your metabolic rate and affect your health in the long term.

Going too long between meals

Are you the type who skips lunch because you're too busy or stressed throughout the day? You may not realize it, but this can set you up to over-eat later on. Eating balanced meals or snacks every 4 hours throughout the day is key to keeping your metabolism working effectively all day long. It also helps keep your blood sugar levels steady so that you're less likely to crash and succumb to cravings, or have poor judgment when it comes to the food decisions you make. To find out more about how blood sugar levels are affected by the foods you eat, refer to Chapter 12.

Breakfast is the most important meal of the day because you're literally breaking your overnight sleeping "fast." Research shows that breakfast jump-starts your metabolism, keeps your energy high, and helps you make healthy decisions all day long. Take a look at Table 2-1 for an example of ideal timing for meals.

Table 2-1	Examples of Ideal Meal Timing
If you wake at 7 a.m.	2 scrambled eggs
Breakfast within 1–2 hours (8–9 a.m.)	1 slice whole wheat toast
	¾ cup berries
	6 ounces nonfat Greek yogurt
Lunch 12–1 p.m.	1 whole wheat pita
	1 cup garbanzo beans
	1 ½ cup spinach salad, cucumber, tomato
	1–2 tablespoons olive oil and vinegar
Snack 4–5 p.m.	4 ounces cottage cheese
	1 apple
	10 almonds
Dinner 8–9 p.m.	3–6 ounces salmon
Bedtime 11 p.m.	1 small baked sweet potato
	1 cup cooked broccoli, zucchini, carrots

Not hydrating enough

You may have heard that drinking more water can help you lose weight. But did you know water can help keep your metabolism moving? About 55–60 percent of your body weight is water, and you lose it through sweat, urination, and respiration. Although your body is smart at regulating the amount you need in order to keep your body temperature stable, eventually you need to drink up to make sure your cells are hydrated adequately. Research shows that when you're dehydrated, your cellular functions slow down. Because on the inside, your body isn't working the best it can, without enough water, you experience fatigue both mentally and physically.

How do you stay hydrated? The old 8×8 rule — eight 8-ounce glasses of water per day — is somewhat outdated. In 2004, The Institute of Medicine (IOM) released adequate intake daily recommendations of 91 ounces for women and 125 ounces for men. These numbers are meant to reflect total water intake, including about 80 percent from beverages, including caffeinated ones, and 20 percent of fluids from foods. Keep in mind that your needs will vary greatly, depending on factors such as exercise, the climate where you live, and how much you sweat. Many do not get the water they need. Here are tips on how to do so:

✔ **Drink at least 20 ounces with meals, 8 ounces with snacks:** Or carry water with you to drink every 1–2 hours throughout the day. Pay attention to when your body feels thirsty; at the first signs, it's telling you that you're already about 2 percent dehydrated. Also, it is common to confuse thirst with hunger, so it's important to stay hydrated to prevent overeating.

✔ **Is drinking plain water unappealing?** Add lemon or cucumber slices for flavor, or one of the all-natural water enhancers on the market. In general, skip sports drinks because they contain added sugar (they can be helpful for athletes exercising at high intensity for 60+ minutes).

✔ **Choose foods with high water content:** It's not called watermelon for nothing. Fruits like melons and veggies like leafy greens contain a large percentage of water that help you get a dose of hydration plus additional valuable vitamins and minerals.

✔ **Replace your fluids:** When exercising, you want to make sure you're hydrating properly to keep your energy high. Aim to drink about 8–10 ounces every 15 minutes. If you're working out intensely, weigh yourself before and after you exercise and drink 16 ounces for every pound lost through sweat.

> ✔ **Alcohol in moderation**: Drinking alcohol can be dehydrating and can also affect your body's ability to metabolize food. When you drink alcohol, your liver works on breaking down alcohol first before any nutrients. If you choose to drink, do so in moderation, which means 1 drink per day for women, 2 for men.

Factoring In Exercise and Stress

Americans are more sedentary than ever before, doing less physical activity and spending more time in front of the computer or television. We also are working longer hours in the office, using more technology, and taking passive modes of transportation (instead of walking or biking, we can take the train or bus), which all add up to less exercise. Less exercise means less calories burned and less muscle mass retained, especially as you age.

Even just making small changes in your routine to boost your activity level can increase your metabolic rate. Try waking up 20 minutes early to take a walk around the neighborhood or make taking the stairs at work the norm — every bit adds up!

Exercise not only helps burn more calories, but also can reduce stress levels. You may be more willing to change your diet than to start an exercise routine, but they're *both* important pieces of the maximizing metabolism puzzle. Doing a combination of cardio and strength training is great, but finding what is realistic for your lifestyle is ideal. For more information on workouts to fit into your day, see Chapter 11.

Your body's response to stress can be harmful to your health and actually cause you to gain weight. From daily stressors, to lack of sleep, to the physical danger of inflammation in your body from disease, your hormone levels can get out of whack and result in a sluggish metabolism. Although you may not be able to eliminate or even control all the sources of stress in your life, you can work on strategies to improve the way your body responds to that stress. Check out Chapter 4 for more information on stress and sleep deprivation.

One sure-fire way to set yourself up for success in boosting your metabolism is to get enough sleep — at least 7 hours per night.

Not only does lack of sleep affect your energy levels and judgment about making healthy choices, it also affects those hormones that regulate your appetite. So you run the risk of overeating on top of an already sluggish metabolism that can result from sleep deprivation.

How Metabolism Affects Physical and Mental Health

It may already be clear to you that as you've aged, your metabolism has slowed down a bit, and maintaining a healthy weight is harder. Maybe when you were younger you never gave a second thought about what you ate, and now you feel you have to be meticulous about every morsel that passes your lips or you'll gain weight.

Following a too-restrictive diet can actually backfire on you, causing your metabolism to slow and making it more difficult to maintain a healthy weight in the long haul. That's why you need to pay attention to additional signs to make sure you're treating your body well. The next section explores how being overweight and obese increases your risk for disease, which can greatly affect your quality of life in many ways. In addition, I outline how to diagnose a sluggish metabolism by how you look and feel.

Body weight and disease

If you're taking in more calories than you're burning, you will gain weight. The Law of Thermodynamics governs the fact that calories in versus calories out regulates body weight. Not sure what a healthy body weight for your height is? To get a general idea, use the Hamwi Method:

For men: 106 lbs. for the first 5 feet + 6 lbs. for each inch over (+/- 10%)

For women: 100 lbs. for the first 5 feet + 5 lbs for each inch over (+/- 10%)

This means if you're a 5'5" woman, your ideal body weight range is 125 pounds, plus or minus 10 percent of the total depending on the size of your frame (subtract 10 percent for a relatively small frame, add it for a relatively large frame). If you're less than 5 feet tall, you can divide the starting number — either 100 or 106 depending on your sex — by 60 inches and then multiply by your height in inches.

Calculating your body mass index or BMI is another general measurement that gives you an idea whether you're within a healthy weight range:

$$BMI = (Weight\ lbs./\ height\ inches^2) \times 703$$

Table 2-2 can help you interpret your BMI.

Table 2-2	BMI chart
BMI	*Range*
< 18.5	Underweight
18.5–24.9	Normal Weight
25–29.9	Overweight
30 >	Obese

The BMI calculation is limited mainly because it doesn't take into account body fat percentage or body shape. If you have a lot of muscle mass, it's possible you can have a high BMI but not be at risk for increased disease. Another measurement, the waist-to-hip ratio, can be used to determine the presence of abdominal obesity and also takes into account body shape. Measure your waist at your belly button and divide that by the measurement of your hips around the middle of your buttocks. A waist-to-hip ratio greater than 0.9 for men or above 0.85 for females is considered abdominal obesity by the World Health Organization. Even in people who are not overweight, a high waist-to-hip ratio can be a risk factor for diabetes, high cholesterol, and high blood pressure.

In 2012, researchers at The City College of New York developed a new obesity measurement tool called A Body Shape Index or ABSI. It combines both waist circumference and BMI to even further delineate body fat percentage and the risks of being overweight. The tool needs further research before use in clinical practice. To learn about the tools that measure your body fat percentage and metabolic rate, refer to Chapter 3.

Type 2 diabetes

About 80 percent of those diagnosed with Type 2 diabetes are overweight or obese. When you're overweight, it becomes more and more difficult for insulin to regulate your blood glucose levels, so your body starts overproducing insulin. Having too much circulating insulin can slow your metabolism even further, which makes your cells even less receptive to taking up blood glucose, known as *insulin resistance*. You can also develop pre-diabetes as your body starts having more trouble regulating blood glucose.

You're more likely to develop diabetes if you have a family history of it, are older than 40, are inactive, and have high blood pressure. Go to your doctor if you're experiencing any of these symptoms related to diabetes:

- ✔ Frequent urination
- ✔ Thirst
- ✔ Blurred vision
- ✔ Cuts and bruises that are slow to heal
- ✔ Fatigue and irritable mood

Heart disease

Carrying too much extra weight also has a negative impact on your circulating lipoprotein and triglyceride levels, which increases your risk for a heart attack, stroke, or other cardiac event.

Hypertension

Your blood pressure increases along with your body weight, which also elevates your risk for heart disease, stroke, and kidney disease. Losing weight can directly result in lowered blood pressure.

Metabolic syndrome

This syndrome is one of the fastest-growing obesity-related concerns in America, and it is classified by a cluster of symptoms like insulin resistance, hypertension, and dyslipidemia. According to the National Health and Nutrition Examination Survey (NHANES), almost a quarter of Americans have this syndrome which puts them at a greater risk of developing the above diseases.

PCOS

This is the most common hormonal disorder among reproductive-age women. It can result in insulin resistance, which makes it a major risk factor for developing diabetes. Most people who develop PCOS are overweight, and it's characterized by an overgrowth of underdeveloped follicles in the ovaries which results in irregular menstrual cycles, ovarian cysts, and excessive hair growth.

Certain cancers

Obesity is correlated with the development of certain types of cancers, such as esophageal, pancreatic, liver, breast, kidney, thyroid, uterine, and colon cancer. Because overall inflammation in the body is also greater when you're overweight, your body is primed for the initiation of tumors. In addition, fat cells release more estrogen, lipase, and additional hormones which may increase tumor growth.

Osteoarthritis

Being overweight puts more pressure than necessary on your joints, making movement more difficult, causing the breakdown of cartilage and the potential need for a joint-replacement surgery. When you're obese, having any type of surgery increases the risk for complications and a longer stay in the hospital.

Sleep apnea

Being overweight can compromise your respiratory function, making it more difficult to get a good night's sleep. Not getting a good night's sleep can in turn increase the risk for obesity, affecting your hormone levels and appetite. See Chapter 3 for more on the effects of sleep deprivation.

I understand it's overwhelming and a little scary to look at these conditions that can accompany having a slow metabolism and carrying too much excess weight. However, it's important to be aware that how you treat your body can have serious consequences in the future. Looking at the big picture of how diet, weight, disease, stress, activity, and sleep all factor in can be a powerful motivator to make change. Go for regular annual check-ups with your physician to monitor your health.

Many nutritionists and doctors will recommend that you start out with a goal of losing just 10 percent of your body weight, at a rate of 1–2 pounds per week. Research shows that even that amount can reduce blood pressure, insulin resistance, and cholesterol levels. Once you succeed with that, you can focus on the next 10 percent, and the next 10, and so on until you're at your ideal body weight. Instead of placing a hyper focus on your ultimate goal, take everything in steps. That way, it will be more manageable, and you'll be more likely to stick to it.

Sick and tired of feeling sick and tired

Although being overweight and having unhealthy habits can result in a disease diagnosis over time, what about day to day? Maybe your metabolism is slowing down for the first time in your life, and risk for disease isn't something that can motivate you to make healthier changes. Perhaps you aren't overweight and just want to break unhealthy habits because you're sick and tired of feeling sick and tired?

When I was a teenager, I became a vegetarian. You might think that translated into a healthier lifestyle, but at that time the quality of my diet was the worst it has been in my life. I actually ate less whole foods, more processed, baked goods and fried foods, and definitely not enough protein. All this took a toll on my digestion, appearance, mood, energy levels, and health. I was always coming down with colds. My mother had the insight to send me to a nutritionist who explained the connection — and I had found my calling in life.

When you're not eating enough and/or not getting the nutrients you need, your body isn't working at peak performance. You've probably experienced one or more of the following symptoms at one point in your life due to unhealthy habits and a sluggish metabolism:

- ✔ **Your energy level is low:** If your metabolism is slow, so is the process of breaking down food and nutrients for energy. So whether you're undereating in general or overeating the wrong types of foods, your energy levels will suffer, and you'll experience fatigue.

- ✔ **Your immune system is weak:** Without getting the nutrients you need, you'll be more likely to take sick days. Your body just isn't as strong as it needs to be to fight off disease. Being inactive, or not getting plenty of exercise, is correlated with a lowered platelet level (*platelets* protect you when a foreign virus or bacteria enters your body).

- ✔ **Your digestion is out of whack:** Without plenty of fiber, movement, and water in your lifestyle, your digestive system won't be working as best it can. You'll experience constipation, bloating, and reflux because your metabolism isn't churning away at the food you eat the way it should be and isn't absorbing it properly for use.

- ✔ **Your mood is depressed:** Not eating balanced meals due to a busy work schedule or stress or any other lifestyle barrier can serve to make you irritable and depressed due to fluctuations in blood sugar. Purposefully depriving yourself and not being satisfied will only leave you cranky and vulnerable to food cravings.

- ✔ **Your mind is foggy:** Your brain requires the right types of nutrients for memory, concentration, and overall alertness. Without it, your resolve to eat better and exercise can diminish, and your judgment isn't as great to make the next right decision when it comes to healthy lifestyle choices.

- ✔ **You aren't as mobile:** If you're overweight and experience joint pain, it may be difficult for you to move around. I'm not only talking about going to the gym for a workout — even day to day tasks can be daunting. Aside from weight, if your energy levels are low, getting motivated to exercise is more difficult, which in turn also affects other pieces of the puzzle, such as mood and digestion.

A slow metabolism doesn't only affect how you feel on the inside. What you put into your body gets broken down and affects your appearance. Although it's not necessarily true that eating too much sugar or fatty foods will cause your skin to break out, those foods are probably replacing more healthful ones in your diet. If you're not getting enough good nutrition because you're depriving your body, not drinking enough water but drinking plenty of alcohol, or not sleeping well, that has an impact on how you look on the outside. Your skin, hair, and nails are constantly regenerating, so if you aren't providing your body with the nutrients for adequate growth, their appearance will be compromised. Outwards signs of a slow metabolism and unhealthful diet include:

✔ Dry, dull, hair or hair loss

✔ Dry, brittle nails

✔ Dry, oily, itchy, discolored or pale skin and acne

✔ Intolerance of cold

Looking at the entire picture of physical and mental health can provide insight into your metabolism and your so-called healthy lifestyle. If you think you're eating nutritiously but experience any of the preceding symptoms, it may be time to reevaluate your plan.

The benefits of making changes in your lifestyle

Do you need more convincing about making changes to your lifestyle? You may be contemplating taking action but aren't ready to make a commitment yet. Maybe up until this point, you've thought it would be too difficult, too costly, or not worth the trouble. You can make changes that will be realistic and sustainable for you, instead of another quick-fix diet or expensive plan that you can't maintain. If you haven't yet realized that diet fads are ultimately damaging to your health, please go back and read Chapter 1. Believe me, I know it's hard to break out of the diet mentality. But the more you learn about metabolism, the more you learn that you can lead a healthy lifestyle without deprivation, with fulfillment, and for the long haul.

Living better

When I worked primarily with eating disorder patients, I saw how dieting, exercising, and weight could dictate someone's life. Both being too restrictive and overeating usually indicate using food for other reasons besides physical hunger. At one point or another, you've probably eaten out of stress, anger, maybe even happiness — in a celebratory manner. But food and emotions are separate, and eating that tub of ice cream doesn't cure your stress. In fact, it will stack feelings of guilt and shame on top of your stress.

On the boosting metabolism plan, the key goal is achieving a balance so that you eat nutritious foods but also allow for fun foods so that you feel satisfied both physically and mentally. You learn to reduce stress without turning to food. You learn how to be active, sleep the best you can, and become more in tune with hunger cues. You eat to live, not the other way around. This all has positive effect on your energy, mood, and quality of life.

Living longer

When you start eating better, exercising, and losing weight, you reduce your risk for obesity and related diseases. Although the life expectancy of the American population is rising due to technology and medical advances, it still lags behind other developed countries. Some researchers believe that the continued uptick in life expectancy will come to an abrupt halt due to the obesity epidemic.

It's never too late to make changes to improve your health, and that's our goal here. So keep your head up and take pride in the fact that each small change you make can add up to big results in the long run.

Chapter 3

Determining and Influencing Your Metabolic Rate

*T*he term *metabolic rate* might be mysterious to you. What does it mean and is it something you can easily measure, like taking your temperature with a thermometer? Not exactly.

Metabolic rate is the pace at which your body digests food and uses the heat that's released for energy. Or more simply: It's the number of calories your body burns. That's why another term for metabolic rate is *burn rate*.

This chapter reviews the equations and procedures that can help you measure your metabolic rate. Your body, your organs, and your involuntary movements (the ones you're not conscious of) all require calories to function, so your burn involves much more than workouts at the gym. You burn calories when you sleep, as you read this book, even while you're eating and taking calories in.

Speaking of eating, one of the main reasons knowing your burn rate is helpful is so you can determine the amount of calories you need to eat to lose, gain, or maintain your weight. Everyone's metabolism moves differently, but certain behaviors and habits can impact your basic needs. This chapter tells you what they are so you can gear up to break those unhealthy habits for good.

You may think of metabolic rate as the speed at which you're able to lose weight. That's a factor, but it's certainly not the entire picture. Your metabolism is like a watermill that requires water (calories) to keep moving and power other processes. You need to burn calories to breathe, keep all your organs in good shape, move, digest, and even just to think. There are many moving parts to the system, each requiring care and attention to function well.

The Lowdown on Metabolic Rate

This section goes over what your metabolic rate is, how to calculate it, and how to test it using various methods. Then you'll be able to estimate what your calorie and nutrient needs are to achieve your goal — whether that goal is losing weight, improving your energy, preventing disease, being active, or just getting the nutrients you need for your health and setting a good example for your children.

Defining metabolic rate

Metabolic rate, as you know, is the rate at which your body burns calories. You can separate the types of calories your body burns into two categories:

- ✔ Resting calories
- ✔ Activity calories

While you're just sitting on your couch or at your desk working, your body is burning a certain amount of baseline calories. This is your body at rest. In fact, the calories your body uses for basic biological functions at rest account for about 60–75 percent of the total amount of energy you burn. While muscle mass burns more than fat mass, your organs use up most of the calories you need for breathing, heart beating, regulating body temperature, digestion, and so on. Table 3-1 breaks down your organs' use of calories (based on estimates by M. Elia in *Organ and Tissue Contribution to Metabolic Weight* [Raven Press, 1992]).

Table 3-1	Energy Expenditure Breakdown by Organ	
Organ	*Select Functions*	*% Expenditure*
Liver	Processing and storing energy, fighting infections, clearing blood of drugs/toxins	27
Brain	Controlling thought, memory, motor actions, senses, every action that regulates the body	19
Heart	Pumping oxygen-rich blood to all cells	7
Kidneys	Filtering system	10
Skeletal muscle	Moving the body	18
Other organs	Performing all other internal functions	19

Several scientific terms can tell you the amount of calories you're burning at rest. I use resting metabolic rate, or RMR.

Although RMR accounts for the majority of calories your body burns, another 25–40 percent of calories are being expended on a daily basis. This energy is called *thermogenesis*. It's the energy used for things like eating, walking around the block, and competing in a triathlon. Adding together RMR and thermogenesis make up the Total Energy Expenditure (TEE), or your total burn rate.

There are three types of thermogenesis:

- ✔ **Exercise thermogenesis:** Physical or daily activities like going to the gym
- ✔ **Non-exercise activity thermogenesis:** Non-structured activity, like shivering or fidgeting
- ✔ **Diet-induced thermogenesis or the Thermic Effect of Food:** Calories burned when breaking down food as you eat it

Depending on how active you are, exercise and movement account for about 15–30 percent of your burn, with about 10 percent from chewing, swallowing, digesting, absorbing, and storing the food you eat. Your body is constantly burning food, which releases units of heat (known as calories but technically called kilocalories, shortened to kcal).

The Law of Thermodynamics states that energy isn't created or destroyed. It is simply transferred from the food you eat to the fuel your body uses to function.

If you aren't eating enough, your body senses deprivation and says, "Hold on. I'm not going to burn if you're not going to eat." That's why your metabolism slows when your diet isn't giving you all the nutrients/calories you need. *Adaptive thermogenesis* is your body's way of protecting you from losing too much energy if you're suddenly dropped onto a desert island. Then when you eat regularly or too much, your body would tend to hold on to those calories because it thinks you're still on a desert island and you're just having a rare feast.

Part of maximizing your metabolism involves ensuring that your body *doesn't* feel deprived so that it keeps on burning calories as effectively as possible.

The degree to which your body burns calories varies based on many factors like what's on your plate and what your diet's been like in the past. Not all calories are created equal either: Protein has a greater *thermic effect* than fat, for example, meaning protein burns faster. Not only does fat give you more calories per gram (9 calories per gram compared to carbs and protein offering 4 calories per gram), but fewer of those calories will be burned through the thermic effect.

Protein really stokes your metabolic fire and keeps it going all day long. I expand on this in Chapter 5.

To actually measure the amount of heat you've lost — to measure your metabolic rate — is a very expensive and complicated procedure. So, most scientists use something called *indirect calorimetry* instead, which measures oxygen consumption and carbon dioxide production. The oxygen you breathe in helps fuel your furnace, as it does when it keeps a fire burning. For each liter of oxygen you take in, a certain amount of calories are expended, and your respiratory exchange ratio (ratio of carbon dioxide to oxygen) determines that amount. The next section discusses methods to calculate your rate based on this measurement.

Calculating metabolic rate

The most basic way to estimate RMR is to use the Mifflin-St Jeor equation. This equation, derived in 1990, came about from measuring indirect calorimetry in human subjects. As far as energy expenditure equations go, it's currently the most accurate, although it has limitations and is normally used as a starting-off point. Mifflin-St Jeor ousted the previously popular Harris-Benedict equation, which was created in 1919 and overestimates RMR by 5 percent.

The Mifflin-St Jeor Equation is as follows, for ages 19–78:

Men: $10 \times$ weight (kg) $+ 6.25 \times$ height (cm) $- 5 \times$ age (y) $+ 5$

Women: $10 \times$ weight (kg) $+ 6.25 \times$ height (cm) $- 5 \times$ age (y) $- 161$

To give yourself an idea of the total calories you're burning in a day, you take that number and multiply it by your personal activity factor:

Sedentary = 1.2

Lightly active = 1.375

Moderately active = 1.550

Very active = 1.725

Extra active = 1.9

If you're like most Americans, you need to convert your weight and height to metric units before entering into the equation:

> ✔ For your weight in kilograms, divide your weight in pounds by 2.2: For example, if you weigh 165 pounds, divide by 2.2 to get 75 kg.

> ✔ For your height in centimeters, multiply your height in inches by 2.54: If you're 5'5", or 65 inches, multiply by 2.54 to get 165.1 cm.

For example, if you're a 45 year-old woman, you'd calculate your RMR like this:

$$(10 \times 75kg) + (6.25 \times 165.1) - (5 \times 45) - 161 = 750 + 1{,}032 - 225 - 161 = 1{,}396 \text{ calories}$$

Then, you'd multiply by your activity factor, which takes into account your day-to-day movement and planned exercise:

> ✔ **If you're sedentary** (you work at a desk job and do very little exercise or housework): $1{,}396 \times 1.2 = 1{,}675$ calories

> ✔ **If you're lightly active** (you go for long walks 1–3 days per week or do housework like cleaning and gardening): $1{,}396 \times 1.375 = 1{,}920$ calories

> ✔ **If you're moderately active** (you're moving most of the day and/or exercise with a moderate amount of effort 3–5 days of the week): $1{,}396 \times 1.550 = 2{,}164$ calories

> ✔ **If you're very active** (you're vigorously exercising or playing sports most days): $1{,}396 \times 1.725 = 2{,}408$ calories

> ✔ **If you're extra active** (vigorous exercise or sports 6–7 days of the week plus a job which requires physical exertion): $1{,}396 \times 1.9 = 2{,}652$ calories

Your turn: What is your total energy expenditure? _____

As you can see, the more active you are, the higher your metabolic rate, or TEE, and the more calories you need. That's why exercise is such a key component of the maximizing your metabolism plan. Even better, the more muscle mass you build, the higher your RMR will be. That's why you want to refer to Chapter 11 to start getting your move on as well.

You wouldn't be crazy to think: "What's the point of changing my diet? If I exercise enough, it won't matter." Unfortunately, unless you're an elite athlete, simply adding exercise won't automatically translate into an increased metabolic rate. Research published July 2012 in the journal *PLos One* examined the Hadza people from Tanzania who are hunter-gatherers. You'd think because they're always active, walking miles and miles every day, that their metabolic rates would be higher. This study found that although their activity was greater than the average Westerner, their metabolic rates were not.

If you eat more than you need, even with additional exercise you can still pack on the pounds. Also, it's possible your body gets used to the type of activity you do on a daily basis, which is why it's important to mix up your exercise routine with strength and interval exercises to keep your body guessing. See Chapter 11 for more.

The Mifflin-St Jeor equation takes into account variables that affect metabolic rate across the board. However, if you're taller, heavier, and more active, you'll burn more calories than a shorter, thinner, less active person. The older you are, the fewer calories you burn due to decrease in muscle over time. And if you're a man, you burn more calories at rest than a woman due to a greater percentage of muscle mass. What the Mifflin-St Jeor equation fails to take into account is variations in individual lifestyle and body composition, meaning you might have different caloric needs than your female friend who is also 5'5", 165 pounds, 45 years old and goes to the same exercise class as you. However, it's a great jumping-off point to start understanding your daily calorie burn.

Measuring metabolic rate and body fat percentage

You can also get your metabolic rate measured using a machine in your doctor's office or at a special laboratory. These types of tests take into account your RMR using indirect calorimetry and also estimate the amount you burn through additional activity based on your height, weight, and the amount of exercise you self-report that you do every day. For best results, you're typically asked to fast overnight and refrain from exercise for 48 hours before engaging in such tests.

How does it work? You breathe into a mouthpiece to calculate your respiratory exchange ratio (RER), and after about ten minutes, you get an estimate. It's not an exact science, but can certainly give you an idea of your total burn rate for the day. Using your RER, you can calculate the calories your body needs and how to adjust this number based on whether you want to lose, gain, or maintain weight.

Related to measuring metabolic rate is measuring your body fat percentage. Because the number on the scale doesn't take into account how much fat versus muscle tissue you have, measuring your body fat percentage helps determine your fitness level. It can be a great tracker to measure your progress as you start maximizing your metabolism.

Yes, your body composition is partially genetic, but most of your fat mass has accumulated over time because of your diet or a sedentary lifestyle. As you start eating a more balanced diet and making time for movement, you can improve your body composition and overall health.

Measuring metabolism on the go

In 2013, four PhDs mostly based out of Arizona State University created a mobile tracking device called Breezing, which measures metabolism when you're out and about. It uses indirect calorimetry to arrive at your RMR, so you can estimate not only how many calories you're burning at rest but also whether you're burning fat, carbs, or a mix of both, depending on your activity level. The device is still in development at the time of writing, but may be shipping by the time you read this. Find out more about Breezing at `http://breezing.co`. (For more on how activity impacts your metabolism, see Chapter 11.)

Here are a few methods for measuring body fat percentage:

- ✔ **Underwater weighing:** Also known as *hydrostatic weighing*, this is when a person is weighed submerged in water. Because lean tissue is denser than fat tissue (remember, muscle weighs more than fat), someone with more body fat will weigh less in water. This method has been known as the "gold standard." In college, I actually did this during class in the basement of our main nutrition building. However, you won't find a water submersion tank just anywhere, and better, more convenient technology (such as DEXA and BodPod, discussed below) will probably become the new gold standard.

- ✔ **Skinfold measurement:** You're more likely to have had this type of measurement performed during an initial fitness test at your gym. This is when your trainer uses calipers on various parts of your body to measure fat thickness. Those measurements are plugged into an equation to estimate your body fat percentage. If done correctly by a well-trained tester, these measurements can be up to 98 percent accurate and are a good way to track changes.

- ✔ **Bioelectrical impedence:** Some scales on the market now not only give you your weight, but also send an electrical current through your body (don't worry, you don't even feel it, and it's completely safe). That current moves differently through fat and fat-free mass, so it can give you an estimation of your fat mass.

- ✔ **DEXA scan:** Used mainly for bone mineral density in medical settings, a dual-energy X-ray absorptiometry (DEXA) measures body composition with considerable accuracy in most situations.

- ✔ **BodPod:** Increasing in popularity, the BodPod works similarly to hydrostatic weighing to measure body composition. However instead of measuring using water, it measures air displacement.

Any type of body testing you do — whether it's getting on the scale in the morning, measuring your body fat percentage at the gym, or getting a metabolic test at your doctor's office — is affected by factors such as your hydration level, what you've eaten, your body temperature, and the hair products you use (just kidding on that last one). Therefore, try to get any kind of testing performed in the same conditions every time to be consistent and to be accurate as a way to track changes.

It's not hard to get obsessed with weighing yourself, but your weight will fluctuate day to day, based on many factors. I recommend that my clients only weigh themselves once a week, on the same day, in the morning before they've eaten or had anything to drink. For some measurements in a medical setting, you're typically asked to wait a few months between tests.

If you have hormone-disrupting condition like hypothyroid, diabetes, or PCOS, or if you've lost a significant amount of weight in the past, research shows that your metabolic rate can be up to 25 percent lower than average. Check with your doctor to see whether getting a metabolic screening test is right for you. Table 3-2 lists select conditions in which your metabolic rate might be significantly altered — either you are hypometabolic (sluggish metabolism with a lower energy expenditure) or hypermetabolic (higher energy expenditure than average). I expand on some of these conditions that cause a lower than normal metabolic rate in Chapter 12.

Table 3-2	Abnormal Metabolic Rate Conditions
Hypometabolic	*Hypermetabolic*
Diabetes	Infection or burns
PCOS	Cancer
Hypothyroid	Hyperthyroid
Cushing's Syndrome	Post-surgery or injury
Grave's Disease	Cirrhosis
Hashimoto's Disease	Prolonged steroid therapy
Anorexia during periods of starvation	Anorexia during refeeding

If you're keeping score at home, you can also use the following equation, which, according to a study in the *British Journal of Nutrition*, can accurately estimate body fat percentage in adults. The equation uses your BMI (or Body Mass Index — for more on what that measurement means, see Chapter 2):

Women: $(1.20 \times BMI) + (0.23 \times Age) - 5.4$

Men: $(1.20 \times BMI) + (0.23 \times Age) - 16.2$

Remember, you can calculate your BMI by dividing your weight in pounds by your height in inches squared and multiply by 703. So continuing with the example of a woman who is 5'5", 165 pounds, and 45 years old, her calculations would look like this:

BMI $= 165 \div 4{,}225 \times 703 = 27.5$

Body Fat Percentage $= (1.20 \times 27.5) + (0.23 \times 45) - 5.4 = 38\%$

Your turn: What is your body fat percentage? _____

Although having too body fat much can increase your risk for obesity-related disease, having too little can be dangerous too. The body needs fat for many functions, such as providing energy, cushioning the organs and tissues, regulating body temperature, and absorbing fat-soluble vitamins such as A, D, E, and K.

Table 3-3 can help you find a normal body fat percentage for you (the data comes from the American Council on Exercise). If you fall below the essential fat cut-off or above the acceptable range, it's time to make changes in your diet and activity. Also note, women have about 5 percent more fat than men — the price we pay to be able to carry and nurture an unborn fetus.

Table 3-3	Body Fat Percentage*	
Classification	**% for Women**	**% for Men**
Essential	10–13	2–5
Athlete	14–20	6–13
Fitness	21–24	14–17
Acceptable	25–31	18–24
Obese	32 and over	25 and over

According to the American Council on Exercise

If your BMI is higher than 25, and you also have a high body fat percentage, don't fret! It's never too late to improve these numbers, boost your health, and maximize your metabolism.

Researchers have made a distinction between where you carry your fat (have you heard of apple and pear shaped?) as having different impact on your risk for health. It's possible that having more abdominal fat (or apple-shaped) means being a greater risk factor for developing diabetes, heart disease, and hypertension. Belly fat is an indicator you are carrying too much fat, but no matter how you cut it (or where you carry it), excess fat is bad for your health. Check out *Belly Fat for Dummies* (Wiley, 2012) for more info about how to banish belly fat.

Not only does a higher body fat composition mean risk for disease, but on a more basic level, fat burns off about one third fewer calories than muscle pound for pound. Fat burns around 3 calories per pound, and muscle about 10 calories per pound. Muscle is a protein powerhouse, and protein synthesis and degradation accounts for about 20 percent of your total RMR. Therefore, by strength training and getting the nutrients/protein you need, you can build and keep those muscles working for you to burn calories so that you lose weight in the form of fat.

How now, brown ... fat?

Researchers have been studying *brown fat* for decades. This is a type of fat that burns large amount of calories to generate heat. Until recently, brown fat was thought to only exist in rodents and infants — to stay warm, because they haven't refined their shiver mechanism. However, in 2009, studies published in the *New England Journal of Medicine* concluded that brown fat does exist in small amounts in human adults, too, and becomes activated in cold temperatures. Your ordinary fat is white, and brown fat is brown because it's composed of mitochondria, those units where energy is produced in cells. When brown fat has used up its own repository for heat, it can actually start working on using your ordinary fat to burn for energy.

People who are thinner and younger have more brown fat than their heavier, older counterparts. So is it the key to a faster metabolism? Should you run out and get a fat transplant? Not exactly. We're a long way off from knowing how brown fat works in humans or whether having more of it would be effective for weight loss. Or if the increased calorie burn would just make us hungrier, causing us to eat more and stay the same weight.

A 2012 study published in *Nature* found that when rats exercise, they release a hormone called irisin, which turns their white fat, brown. Hope for people? Maybe so. People also have irisin in their blood. Just another reason to get your move on with exercises in Chapter 11.

Determining Calorie and Nutrient Needs

One major reason 32 percent of Americans are obese is a disproportionate energy balance — we take in too many calories and burn too few. There are many theories about why that is: changes in food supply, more people dining out, bigger portion sizes, decreased access to healthy foods. Regardless of the reasons, the World Health Organization reports that by 2030, the obesity rate will increase to 42 percent of the U.S. population.

Now that you've got an idea of the total calories you burn every day and what your body fat percentage is, it's time to figure out the amount of calories you need to eat every day.

This is just an estimate. Weight loss is more than just the total number of calories you take in and expend. It involves, among other things, getting enough activity, the timing and composition of meals, how much you sleep, and what you do to relax. That sounds like a lot of work, and, to be frank, it is. But you're going to take steps one at a time. In this section, I go over how you can best fuel your body to continue steadily losing weight.

Using your metabolic rate to establish calorie needs

You may have heard that 3,500 calories is equal to a pound of body weight — so, the less you eat, the more you'll lose. While working at CalorieCount.com where I counsel people online, I've seen first-hand how many don't succeed at losing weight, even knowing this info, because they either don't change their calorie intake as they lose weight or they eat too little overall. They come to a halt or complain that they've hit a *plateau* (which, by the way, is a word that is misused all the time, a topic I return to momentarily).

By reevaluating your meal plan and your goals to make sure they're realistic, and making small tweaks to your meal plan instead of an overhaul, you can stay on the healthy weight loss straight and narrow.

Plateaus are natural and occur because once you've been losing weight for a while, you need to change up your routine. As you lose weight, your metabolism slows, you require fewer calories, you might be losing that oh-so-beneficial muscle mass, and so on. Whatever its cause, remember that a plateau is your body's way of telling you that your metabolism needs a little boost.

Back to that number of 3,500 calories per pound: Although not entirely clear cut, the number is a decent estimation to go by to calculate the nutrients you need. Because a week has 7 days, to lose 1 pound per week, you'd need to cut out 500 calories per day. Want to lose 2 pounds per week? Cut out 1,000 calories per day.

Want to lose 3 pounds per week? Stop right there. A healthy rate of weight loss is 1–2 pounds (0.5-1 kg) per week. Anything greater than that, and you run the risk of adaptive thermogenesis — a significant slowing of your metabolism, loss of muscle mass, and risk for nutrient deficiencies.

To make sure you're getting enough calories but not too many, take your total energy expenditure and subtract about 500-1,000 calories either by eating that much less per day or adding that many to your burn through exercise. For example, let's say you're typically lightly active, and your burn rate is 1,900 calories. You need to do one of the following:

- ✔ Increase your activity level on top of what you are already doing day-to-day
- ✔ Eat 1,200–1,400 calories per day
- ✔ Combine both ways, such as eating 1,500 calories per day and burning an additional 200 through exercise.

Here are the minimum daily calories your body needs at rest to fuel your organs and muscles, according to the American College for Sports Medicine:

- ✔ 1,200 calories for women
- ✔ 1,800 calories for men

These are the absolute minimum calories you should be consuming. If you have more muscle or very active, you need to add more to the baseline. How much more? Basically, you shouldn't exceed a total deficit greater than 1,000 calories. If you eat 1,900 calories, but have a burn of 2,900 calories throughout the day from your RMR plus additional exercise, that would correlate to a –1000 calorie deficit, which is the maximum recommended for healthy weight loss.

The magic number that will work for you may be discovered through trial and error. Some research shows that cutting just 100 calories per day from what you typically eat can have a great effect on health and weight. Your magic number will change as your body changes. (Well, it's not really magic, it's science.)

In 2012, researchers at the National Institute of Diabetes and Digestive and Kidney Diseases created an online tool that predicts how your body composition will change depending on changes in your diet and activity level. You can find the tool at http://bwsimulator.niddk.nih.gov/. It calculates the number of calories you need during weight loss and maintenance phases. You can also enter when you changed your calorie intake and get a prediction for when you'll reach your goal weight. It's a great reminder right off the bat that your needs will evolve throughout the process.

These researchers found that body reaction time was very slow for weight change and that it took three years for someone losing weight to reach their *steady* or maintenance state. Don't let this discourage you; I only mention this so that you keep in mind that this is about making changes for good. You can still take steps so that you look and feel your best for the short term, but realize you are doing so to improve your lifestyle for the long term.

Don't feel like doing any equations or younger than 18 years old? Table 3-4 gives you an idea of the calories you need every day for weight maintenance. If you're older than 18, for 1 pound per week weight gain, add 500 calories per day and 1 pound per week weight loss, subtract 500 calories per day. For people under age 18 years, because you're still growing and developing, it's important that you consult with your physician before starting in with any weight loss plan.

Table 3-4	Estimated Calorie Needs			
Sex	**Age (years)**	**Sedentary**	**Moderately Active**	**Active**
M/F	2–3	1,000	1,000–1,400	1,000–1,400
F	4–8	1,200–1,400	1,400–1,600	1,400–1,800
	9–13	1,400–1,600	1,600–2,000	1,800–2,200
	14–18	1,800	2,000	2,400
	19–30	1,800–2,000	2,000–2,200	2,400
	31–50	1,800	2,000	2,200
	51+	1,600	1,800	2,000–2,200
M	4–8	1,200–1,400	1,400–1,600	1,600–1,800
	9–13	1,600–2,000	1,800–2,200	2,000–2,600
	14–18	2,000–2,400	2,400–2,800	2,800–3,200
	19–30	2,400–2,600	2,600–2,800	3,000
	31–50	2,200–2,400	2,400–2,600	2,800–3,000
	51+	2,000–2,200	2,200–2,400	2,400–2,800

Source: HHS/USDA Dietary Guidelines for Americans 2010. Calorie levels are rounded to the nearest 200 mark.

Table 3-4 doesn't take into account females who are pregnant or lactating. Add 300 calories per day in the second and third trimesters of pregnancy, and 500 calories per day during lactation to these numbers.

Keeping the fire burning

When weight loss results slow or stop, many of my clients get discouraged, think they've failed, and self-sabotage all their healthy efforts. They do this by either going back to eating all junk food, becoming sedentary, or turning to something like a cleanse or crash diet to keep them going.

If this sounds like you, you need to change your mentality — otherwise you're not going to be able to successfully change your behaviors. More on this in Chapter 4.

While you can't stop your metabolism from naturally slowing down a bit as you lose weight, you *can* prevent this process from being too rapid. Otherwise, it's more likely it will be difficult to maintain that weight loss because you haven't given your body proper time to adjust. Your instinct might be for you to restrict too much or turn to a popular very low calorie or low-fat or low-carb diet. The following are some side effects of not getting enough calories and macronutrients — they're meant to scare, I mean educate, you on why you need to fuel and keep your furnace burning:

- ✔ **Calories:** Because a calorie is a unit of energy — literally heat — not getting enough calories can slow your metabolic rate by as much as 30 percent. Your body will start breaking down your beneficial muscle mass for fuel.

- ✔ **Proteins:** Enzymes in proteins make processes of metabolism happen. Enzymes are also building blocks for your hair, nails, and muscles. If you don't get enough proteins, your body has more difficulty building and maintaining that calorie-burning muscle.

- ✔ **Carbohydrates:** Carbohydrates provide energy for your body and brain. Not getting enough of the beneficial carbs can cause you to feel fatigue, be more stressed, and have trouble sleeping — all symptoms that wreak havoc on your metabolic rate.

- ✔ **Fat:** You might be trying to lose fat, but you still need to eat it. Without enough fat, your body can't make enough hormones, including leptin which helps regulate your metabolic rate and appetite.

Any restrictive or fad "diet" that cuts out one of the preceding macronutrients is not providing you the balance that you need to keep your metabolism moving and your energy high. You should discontinue it immediately!

Balancing food quality

As I mention many times throughout this book, balance is key to boosting your metabolism. One aspect of this is to make sure you get a balance of nutrients both throughout the day and within mealtimes. You also want to have a balance of food that tastes good and is good for you, so that you don't feel deprived.

Weight *maintenance* can often be more difficult than weight loss. Why? Because your body requires fewer calories as you lose the weight. That's hard to deal up with in addition to the other changes your body goes through, such as changes in hormones. So make sure that you don't feel deprived, that you are feeding your body what it needs for energy.

Although diets that especially restrict carbohydrates might result in weight loss, research conducted at the New Balance Foundation Obesity Prevention Center at Boston Children's Hospital found that restricting carbs resulted in an increase in cholesterol and other indicators for heart disease and diabetes. A low-fat diet in this study correlated with lowered metabolic rate *plus* these risk factors. The winner was a diet that was a low-glycemic index diet, which emphasized a more even proportion of fat, carbs, and protein.

The *glycemic index* (GI) scale measures how fast and high a food causes your blood sugar to increase. Too fast and high, and your body releases too much insulin to counteract that blood sugar. Too much circulating insulin increases risk for diabetes, high blood pressure, high cholesterol, and obesity. Therefore, foods that have a low GI are more likely to keep your blood sugar levels, and these risk factors, under control. However, the GI of a food is affected by its preparation and what else it's eaten with — that's why I place much more importance on the balance between nutritious sources of macronutrients.

The results of the study at Boston Children's Hospital point out that you can't just think in terms of low fat and low carb. It's the quality of those calories that count! Choose lean proteins, high-fiber carbohydrates, and heart-healthy fats (more on these in Chapter 5). In general, you want proportions that look like this:

- **Carbohydrates:** 45–65 percent of calories
- **Proteins:** 10–35 percent of calories
- **Fats:** 20–35 percent of calories

Table 3-5 compares low-fat, low-carb, and balanced diets, with typical examples of each.

Table 3-5	Comparison of Daily Diets		
Meal	*Low-Fat*	*Low-Carb*	*Balanced*
Breakfast	Sesame bagel with fat-free cream cheese	Eggs, cheese, and bacon	Eggs with whole wheat toast and an orange
Lunch	Grilled chicken over spinach salad, chickpeas, sliced apples, vinegar, and bag of pretzels	Grilled chicken over spinach salad, walnuts, olive oil	Grilled chicken over spinach salad, chickpeas, sliced apples, walnuts, and olive oil
Snack	Low-fat yogurt and dried fruit	Nuts and cheese	Low-fat yogurt and berries
Dinner	Pasta with marinara sauce and broccoli	Sirloin with side iceberg lettuce wedge	Sirloin with baked potato and broccoli

Do any of the meals under the low-fat or low-carb columns look familiar to you in your daily diet? That means you're ready to start incorporating more balance into your meal plan!

Lifestyle Factors That Impact Your Rate

In this chapter you've read about what metabolic rate means, how to calculate it, what that means for your calorie and nutrient needs, and the impact of nutrition on your metabolic rate. But what about other aspects of your lifestyle that could be impacting your ability to burn calories off? How are your habits affecting your metabolic rate?

Not moving enough

I've found in practice that to lose weight, women are more likely to focus on reducing calories, and men are more likely to increase exercise than change their diet. Maybe it's due to stereotypes around each activity. Women don't want to build bulky muscle, so they shy away from the weights completely.

Dieting might seem too feminine for men. I hope by now you can predict what I have to say about this: No matter your gender, you need to focus on *both* to get good results in weight and health.

Recently in the media, the term *skinny fat* has been used to describe celebrities who are at a low to normal weight for their height but don't have any tone or strength to their bodies. I don't particularly like this term but I do like the message behind it. Skinny does not equal healthy. In fact, I'd venture to guess these people's metabolic rates are moving at the pace of a snail. And they may be at increased risk for osteoporosis and heart disease.

Without incorporating activity and strength training, you're missing out on reaping benefits for heart and bone health and disease prevention. In addition, your metabolism won't be as revved if you're just dieting to lose weight and aren't thinking about preserving your lean muscle mass for long-term health. By getting a variety of exercise, you can keep your metabolic rate moving all day long.

Effects of too much stress

We've all been there. Pressure from work deadlines, taking care of your family, dealing with financial struggles or personal loss — Americans are seriously stressed out. Stress can be a big barrier to making healthy lifestyle changes, but it's a double-edged sword: Stress itself can result in a sluggish metabolic rate.

Here's how it works: When you're stressed, your body releases *cortisol*, a hormone that regulates the energy you use and distributes fat within your body. Being stressed over the years, lots of cortisol floating around causes increases in blood sugar and insulin, which become more and more difficult to balance in the body. Cortisol increases your appetite and stores that extra glucose as fat.

Researchers agree that cortisol alone isn't responsible for the U.S. obesity epidemic. However, over time, your body develops more fat storage and more fat mass, which ultimately slows your metabolic rate.

Stress also upsets your digestive system. You might be experiencing stomach issues from too much stress, which could then affect what you eat. When your stomach is bothering you, you may have difficulty eating every 4 hours or choosing high-fiber foods — both of which are strategies to maximize your metabolic rate. So, learning how to relax and deal with your stress more effectively has many benefits.

Effects of sleep deprivation

If you're experiencing stress in your life, your sleep is often affected as well. Either you aren't getting enough good quality sleep because you're tossing and turning, or you have disruptions in sleep because of your weight and respiratory issues. Maybe you just have difficulty powering down at the end of the day or are at work late at night and up early in the morning. Over the past several decades, the amount of sleep Americans get on average has decreased 2 hours per night, from 8.5 hours to 6.5 hours.

Similar to stress, a poor night's sleep — less than 7 hours — can cause you to wake up and go straight for that chocolate iced donut. Your inhibitions are lowered because you haven't properly recharged. Also, you might find yourself eating more throughout the day because you feel like it will help you wake up.

On a more cellular level, research shows that not getting enough sleep directly impacts your hormones that regulate appetite and blood sugar control:

- ✔ **Ghrelin is increased:** Increases appetite and decreases energy expenditure

- ✔ **Leptin is decreased:** Decreases appetite and increases energy expenditure

- ✔ **Insulin is decreased:** Regulates blood sugar

- ✔ **Cortisol is increased:** Promotes fat storage

A good night's sleep is just as important as a healthy day of eating and activity for optimizing your metabolic rate. It also helps keep your risk for diabetes and metabolic syndrome at bay. For more on these hormone-disrupting conditions, see Chapter 12.

Effects of smoking and drinking

Turning to smoking or drinking alcohol as your main stress relief might work in the short term for you, but in the long term they negatively affect your weight and health. This is probably not news to you but let me explain why.

- ✔ **Smoking cigarettes:** In addition to how difficult it is to quit the habit, people might be afraid to quit because nicotine does suppress your appetite, and once you quit, metabolic rate decreases. However, this isn't significant compared to the health risks of smoking such as lung cancer and raising your risk for heart disease. Your metabolic rate can rebound with activity and nutritious eating.

✔ **Drinking alcohol:** In moderation, alcohol might have health benefits, but because your body needs to focus on metabolizing alcohol when it enters your bloodstream, it puts food on the backburner. Also when your liver is working on breaking down alcohol, it decreases the amount of fat your body can use for energy and, therefore, stores it. Overall, drinking alcohol impairs digestion and absorption of vitamins and minerals.

Lifestyle habits you want to pick up include moderate amounts of caffeine and drinking enough water. They've both been shown to increase metabolic rate and keep you energized:

✔ **Drinking water:** Research published in *The Journal of Clinical Endocrinology and Metabolism* suggests that by consuming an extra 1.5 liters (about 34 ounces) of water per day over the course of a year, you could lose 5 pounds due to the increase in metabolic rate and calories burned.

Add ice to your water! Much of the increase in metabolic rate is likely due to your body regulating temperature from drinking water that is cold.

✔ **Drinking caffeine:** Found in coffee, teas, and colas, caffeine has been shown to increase metabolic rate and fat burned. Having 200–300 mg in addition to a nutritious diet might help boost your rate.

Many caffeinated drinks like colas and specialty coffee drinks also contain a lot of refined sugar and saturated fat, which can outweigh the beneficial effects of the caffeine. Also, caffeine can increase anxiety and interfere with a good night's sleep. Keep this in mind as you add caffeine to your day and moderate your amount if you experience these negative effects.

Effects of medication

Prescription medications can potentially affect your metabolic rate. Always consult your physician before discontinuing any medication if it has negative side effects like weight gain. Remember the positive effects of these medications; your doctor should determine whether the risks outweigh the benefits. You may need to change your eating behavior and exercise if you must continue on a particular prescription.

It's also not always clear whether a medicine is resulting in weight gain because of your metabolic rate or whether it's really due to improved appetite or other factors. For instance, an antidepressant might make you regain your appetite which was lost due to depression.

Weight gain from medication can result in serious health conditions like diabetes and metabolic syndrome, so always speak with your doctor about potential side effects. Some medications notorious for weight gain include anti-psychotics for mood disorders, corticosteroids to treat inflammation, and beta-blockers for high blood pressure. Medications as well as lifestyle habits affect everyone differently. Being mindful of this is very important as you make your way down the road to boosting your metabolism and improving your health.

Part II

Laying the Groundwork for Boosting Your Metabolism

Five Small Changes for Big Results

- ✔ Eat breakfast. A balanced breakfast of lean protein and fiber helps start your metabolism engine for the day. If you skip a morning meal, your body proceeds at a more sluggish rate.

- ✔ Go for a 30-minute walk. You don't have to spend hours at the gym to achieve results. Getting moving with just 30 minutes per day can be a realistic way for you to stay motivated and burn calories.

- ✔ Give yourself 30 minutes of me time to do whatever makes you happy. Being stressed affects your hormones and can slow down your metabolic rate. Take time for yourself every day to do an activity that gives you pleasure and is relaxing.

- ✔ Cook dinner instead of dining out. Cooking at home helps take in more metabolism-boosting nutrients and cuts down on hidden sources of sodium, sugar, and saturated fat in many restaurant meals.

- ✔ Choose an extra serving of fruit or vegetables with your meal. Fruits and veggies are packed with fiber which help keep you satisfied.

The *For Dummies* web site for this book offers some great extra goodies on boosting your metabolism — such as how to pick up metabolism-boosting foods at the grocery store. Check it out at www.dummies.com/extras/boostingyourmetabolism/.

In this part . . .

- ✔ Get ready to make changes in diet and behavior that will actually last.

- ✔ Understand the ins and outs of which foods are best for boosting your metabolism.

- ✔ Get the low-down on spices and organic foods and how they affect your metabolism.

- ✔ Figure out what true hunger is and what to do when it's not true hunger.

- ✔ Plan your meals with sample ideas.

Chapter 4

Preparing Your Mind and Body for a Healthier Life

In This Chapter

▶ Getting ready to make changes that will last

▶ Focusing on hindering foods and habits

▶ Putting a successful plan in place

Maybe you woke up this morning and said to yourself, "Today is the day I start my diet." You packed a healthy lunch before heading off to work. When you got into the office, the donut box in the kitchen was an instant reminder that it was your coworker's last day. Everyone else was having one — how could you pass it up? Come lunchtime, the coworker you lunch with had grabbed some pizza and was sitting in the park. You could have brought your sandwich and sat with her, but you thought, "I already had that donut today. I might as well have pizza, too. I'll start my diet tomorrow."

If this anecdote sounds familiar, you're not alone. You *want* to make changes, but life gets in the way, and you always put it off or simply don't know where to start. You may think you know how to live a healthy lifestyle, but it hasn't worked for you in the past. In this chapter, you'll find out step by step how to take action and make your goals a reality.

If there's one thing I want you to take away from this chapter it's to think beyond starting a restrictive "diet." I outline foods and habits you want to limit to maximize your metabolism, but the bottom line is that *unless a plan is realistic for you, it won't be sustainable in the long term.* You can be your own diet detective and identify the foods that have been thwarting your weight loss efforts. I talk about the best ways to boost your metabolism, but more importantly, I tell you how you can plan ahead to incorporate these changes into your lifestyle, track your progress, and stay on a path toward steady weight loss and improved health.

Gearing Up for the Big Change

Before instituting any kind of change in your life, it's important to prepare yourself so that you're more successful with what lies ahead. This means different things for different people, but the first step for most is recognizing there is a problem and being motivated for change. If you're there, then you can start working on your mentality so you're focused and can keep your eye on your end goal. This section reviews the best approach to making the mental changes you need so that you'll more likely achieve the results you want without getting sidetracked.

Starting small for big results

Clients will come into my office and say, "I want to lose 50 pounds. How can I do that?" Or: "I want to compete in a triathlon," but they've never even run a mile. It's great to have big goals to aim for, but overhauling your entire lifestyle all at once can backfire. Having an "all or nothing" mentality can make you feel like you've accomplished nothing, when in fact, you did make a healthy choice that day (for example, if you chose that turkey sandwich over your coworker's pizza). Even if it feels good when you're doing "all," such as sticking to a rigid diet and exercise schedule, you feel guilt or shame when you aren't able to keep it up to perfection. It becomes a vicious cycle because guilt and shame don't motivate you to take positive steps.

Making smaller changes and tweaks to your current eating and exercise habits can be more likely to translate into long-term changes. Because your unhealthy habits developed over many years, you can't break them overnight. Thinking that you can will only lead to frustration. Or if you just feel deprived and fatigued, you'll also feel miserable, and these will certainly not be changes that you can maintain.

There's a great online program called Couch to 5K (www.c25k.com) for beginning runners. It acknowledges that you're not going to wake up and run three miles if you've never been a runner before. It's about taking small steps, day by day, week by week, to reach your goals.

If you think about any exercise or diet program you've tried in the past, it probably emphasized more of the "all or nothing" approach. Sure, it could work in the short term, but not for the long haul — and if you're not eating enough or are over-exercising, it could also have a negative effect on your metabolic rate.

Write down a list of small changes you think you'd be willing to try and incorporate into your lifestyle. Post this list on the inside of your bathroom cabinet or keep it next to your bed for inspiration when you wake up. It can also be a reminder that when things don't go exactly as planned, you can just do the *next* right thing instead of sabotaging your entire day.

Here are some ideas for your list:

- ✔ Eat breakfast
- ✔ Go for a 20-minute walk
- ✔ Swap out a caloric beverage like soda for water
- ✔ Take a 30-minute lunch break and be mindful when eating
- ✔ Swap out white bread for whole wheat bread
- ✔ Have a piece of fruit as part of a snack
- ✔ Give yourself 30 minutes of *me time* to do whatever makes you happy
- ✔ Cook dinner instead of dining out
- ✔ Choose an extra serving of vegetables with your meal
- ✔ Turn off all electronics 30 minutes before bedtime to prepare for a good night's sleep.

Even if you just do one of these things one day per week, you can feel proud of yourself for starting to be more mindful of your health and improving your metabolism. If these items are too basic for you, build upon them to come up with tasks that are challenging but not impractical. For example, increasing amount of days you complete them or amount of time you spend. Or adding more and more to the list as you feel you're able to without feeling overwhelmed.

Avoiding the wrong kind of motivation

If you've started and stopped lots of nutrition and exercise plans — if you can't even remember a time when you weren't trying to change your habits — you need to assess your motivation. Before you can change your behavior, you have to change your thought process. That wasn't part of my dietetics degree curriculum, but later on, I realized how powerful thoughts can really be.

When working with patients who struggle with eating disorders, I've learned a lot from therapists and patients alike about how much of an impact negative thoughts and self-talk can have on behaviors and mood. One example of these negative thoughts is the "all or nothing" (or "black and white") mentality mentioned earlier.

Do you feel like if you aren't doing things *perfectly*, you've failed? With that thought can come feelings of shame, depression, and a reduced motivation to do anything for fear of continued failure. You decide to dip into that bag of chips in the kitchen because you think, "What's the point?" By the time your hand hits the bottom of that bag, you feel even worse about yourself and vow all over again to be *perfect* starting tomorrow.

Believing in this ideal of perfection or a quick-fix for weight loss is unrealistic, irrational, and counter-productive to reaching your goals.

Consider these questions:

- ✔ When you get a compliment from someone, do you jump to the conclusion that they don't really mean it?
- ✔ Do you constantly make *should* statements like "I *should* go to the gym" or "I *shouldn't* eat this" and then feel bad about yourself when you don't do those things?
- ✔ Do you have negative feelings about your body when you look in the mirror?
- ✔ Do you tend to blow your weaknesses out of proportion?

If you responded yes to one or more of those questions, you're using the wrong kind of motivation and are negatively affecting your ability to change.

First you need to be aware of your negative thoughts, and then you need to restructure them. The following are some ideas on how you could change a thought and put a positive twist on it to stop the negativity:

- ✔ **If you don't believe a person is being genuine about a compliment:** What is the evidence that they're not? Could it be that I'm projecting my own negative thoughts, and the person is being sincere?
- ✔ **If you're making too many *should* statements:** Even if it takes more time than I thought, I will make these changes. Maybe I'm not going to the gym because I hate it there, not because I'm a failure. How can I make activity fun?
- ✔ **If you have a low body image:** Would I say any of these negative things to a best friend about their body? What about to a 5-year-old version of myself? What are the things I love about my body? (Make a list: *My blue eyes. My strong, shiny hair.*)
- ✔ **If you exacerbate your weaknesses:** What are my strengths and how can those help me work on and overcome my weaknesses? I have the power to improve myself one step at a time.

I know your negative thoughts are by now automatic, and it's hard to control them because it's the way you've been thinking for a long time. But the more you practice stopping yourself, and the more you come up with other mantras or positive assertions and questions, the more productive you'll be toward attaining your end goal.

Banishing "good" and "bad"

"I'm not eating carbs. Carbs are bad." What does this statement even mean? It totally drives me nuts when people call foods *good* and *bad* because that doesn't offer any specifics. For example, a piece of fruit can be "bad" if it's overripe or rotten; a piece of cake is "good" because that's how it tastes.

Of course, some foods are more nutritious than others, and some stoke your metabolic rate and promote weight loss, but classifying them as *good* and *bad* can affect your psyche. When you eat something that's "bad," you're more likely to feel shame around consuming it — which then makes it a very popular choice for overeating for emotional reasons.

In a similar vein, you may be blindly following a popular fad diet. You heard that you can lose weight on this diet, so you do it without even questioning why some foods are limited while others are included. If you do understand why some foods are more nutritious than others, and you know you consume too much of the food that can be a barrier to reaching your goals, then that's a reason to monitor your consumption of it.

Being so strict with yourself can backfire. If you have a restrictive dieting mentality, you're definitely rolling your eyes at me. I've heard it all before: "How can I lose weight if I allow myself a treat every day?" Well, check this out: A 2012 study at Tel Aviv University found that when people on a low-calorie diet consumed a big breakfast containing a sweet, they lost more weight than those who didn't have a dessert with their morning meal. One reason for this might be because the participants were more satisfied and less likely to experience cravings later in the day. This is just one study, but it contains a germ of truth that I have seen time and time again in clinical practice.

When you completely avoid a food, you're more likely to give in and overeat that food when faced with it down the road. Also, depriving yourself can actually slow your metabolism, leaving you feeling fatigued and reducing your resolve to fight cravings. Allowing yourself to indulge *in moderation* takes away idealization of your forbidden or "bad" foods, so you're less likely to

73

overdo it, especially when vulnerable because of emotions like stress. Be an educated consumer and don't simply dismiss something as "bad" — learn *why* it's not going to help you reach your goals.

Don't give in to peer pressure from friends or family members who aren't willing to change their thought processes. You're doing this for *you*, not for anyone else's approval. Whenever you feel like you might give in to peer pressure — either to revert to a restricting dieting mentality or to eat something you don't need — don't defend yourself to others. Just stay strong in your convictions and remind yourself that you're changing your attitude because nothing else has worked for you in the past. Do that, and you'll develop a healthier relationship with food and yourself.

What to Minimize In Your Diet

When you're motivated to improve your health and boost your metabolic rate, you need to find out about the foods and nutrients that may be thwarting your best efforts. You can start preparing your body for improved health by first realizing where you need to make changes in your own diet in ways that will be realistic for you.

This section outlines the major offenders that stand in your way to a maximized metabolism. Many of these foods are *processed*, meaning they do not occur in nature and have been altered in some way by the food industry before you eat them. The alteration can occur through freezing, canning, dehydration, refrigeration, and so on. The end result can often be a food that's less nutritious than before.

Not all foods that are processed are detrimental to your health. For example, before you drink it, raw milk is pasteurized to kill bacteria that can cause foodborne illness. Another example is frozen produce. Freezing is usually done so at the peak of ripeness so that those fruits and veggies retain optimal nutrition as they are transported and handled, versus fresh fruit which loses nutrients quickly as it becomes overripe.

The first step to reducing the metabolism busters outlined in this section is to remove them from your kitchen cabinets. That way, you won't be tempted to dig in when you're vulnerable due to stress, sadness, happiness, or just boredom when you're sitting around mindlessly eating and watching television.

Beware of synthetic carbs

Often in the dieting community a scapegoat emerges that gets blamed for weight gain. In the mid-1990s, it was fat. And actually a push to decrease dietary fat in the American food supply resulted in an increase in the amount of grain in the food supply. Unfortunately, much of this grain was refined so that it could be used in a wide range of products, for example to improve the texture of food and extend its shelf life. Products containing more and more added sugar also hit the marketplace. These *synthetic carbohydrates* are not nutritious. American's consume too much of them, and they should be seriously reduced in your diet.

Refined grains

When a grain is whole, it contains a germ, bran, and endosperm (see Figure 4-1). When it's refined, the bran and germ are removed — a process that also removes fiber, vitamins, and minerals. B vitamins, iron, and folic acid may be added back in, but not necessarily to the extent that they existed originally. And fiber is typically not added back in at all.

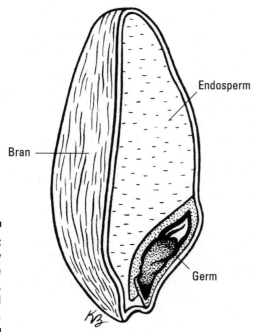

Figure 4-1:
Anatomy of a whole grain: germ, bran, and endosperm.

Illustration by Kathryn Born

Enriched refined grains do offer some nutrition, but the original whole grain contains more nutrients to fuel your body and keep your metabolism moving. Also think about where you may find refined grains. Many of those products often also contain saturated fat, sodium, and other additives. Here are a few of the major sources of refined grains in the American diet:

- ✔ White breads, rice, pastas
- ✔ Tortillas, tacos, and pizza
- ✔ Cakes, cookies, pies, pastries
- ✔ Potato chips, corn chips, pretzels

According to a 2010 survey published in *Journal of the American Dietetic Association*, fewer than 10 percent of Americans consume enough whole grains; refined grains play a major role in most people's diet. This puts you at increased risk for obesity and makes it more difficult to maintain a healthy weight.

I'm not blaming the obesity epidemic on the prevalence of more refined grains (or any one component of lifestyle for that matter) because other factors are at play, such as Americans being more sedentary and the increase in portion sizes over the years. But if you consume more whole grains, you'll be getting less of the stuff you don't want and more real food as it's found in nature — which is the stuff a boosted metabolism is made of.

Products can contain a mix of whole grains and refined grains. To make sure your product contains whole grains, you want one of the *first* ingredients to say whole wheat, whole grain, or whole something else. Ingredients are listed in order of weight. The closer an ingredient is to the top of the list, the more weight it comprises of the product. You can usually spot a refined grain product if the label mentions it's "enriched" and if it contains little fiber. Refined grain products, especially those with added solid fats and sodium, are at the top of your list to minimize.

Added sugars

Here's a fun analogy when it comes to health effects: Whole grains are to refined grains as naturally occurring sugars are to what? The answer is *added sugar*, which makes up the majority of sugar Americans consume. In fact, on average a person in the United States gets about 22 teaspoons of added sugar per day, which adds up to about 330 calories!

Cutting out foods with added sugars, which typically only provide excess calories with little nutrition, can help you lose up to a pound per week.

Natural sugars are found in fruits, as *fructose*, and milk, as *lactose*, and in vegetables and some grains that your body uses for energy. Your body also uses processed sugar for energy, but typically, added (processed) sugars provide calories in excess of what your body needs and so get converted into fat.

Just like whole and refined grains, some products may contain both natural and added sugars. Typically, products which contain sources of milk and fruit have natural sugars but can also have added sugar. Reading a food label, it's hard to tell which of the sugar is coming from natural or added sources. That's why there's a push from the U.S. Food and Drug Administration to get "added sugar" on food labels. Many groups, such as the American Heart Association and the Center for Science in the Public Interest, are behind this effort. The idea is that such information on a label would be helpful for consumers to distinguish between the two kinds of sugar and make more healthful choices.

Added sugar includes what you sprinkle on your cereal or pour in your coffee, but added sugars are also found in so many foods to improve flavor, texture, and appearance. Table 4-1 lists some of these.

Table 4-1	Added Sugars in Common Foods	
Food	*Serving Size*	*Calories from Added Sugar per Serving*
Carbonated soda	12 ounce can	132.5
Lemonade	1 cup	99.2
Cranberry sauce, canned, sweetened	1 slice	86.4
Gumdrop candies	10 each	84.8
Non-fat fruit yogurt	6 ounces	77.5
Milk chocolate	1 bar	77.4
Vanilla ice cream	½ cup	61.2
Granola bar	1	56.0
Banana chips	1 ounce	39.6
Ketchup	1 table-spoon	13.6

Source: From USDA database for the added sugar content of selected food

---

Yet another sugar: Blood glucose

You know now that foods with both refined carbs and added sugars typically add excess calories without the wholesome nutrition found in real, unprocessed foods. However, their effect on your blood sugar, or glucose, levels can also be detrimental to your health.

Because these processed foods often don't contain fiber but rather simple sources of carbohydrate, they cause a rapid spike in your blood sugar levels and a rapid release of insulin, which scurries to try to get that blood sugar absorbed into your cells. Over time, your cells become desensitized to that insulin, which is known as *insulin resistance*, and that can lead to an increase in your risk for diabetes.

 Although there isn't an "added sugar" row yet on a Nutrition Facts label, you can read through the ingredients to see if there is added sugar in the product. Remember the closer to the top of the list, the heavier the weight of that sugar, so you're able to at least get a feel for the amount the product contains.

Sugar sneaks in under these names on labels:

- ✔ Anything ending in –*ose*: Dextrose, sucrose, maltose, lactose, fructose
- ✔ Syrup, corn syrup, and high fructose corn syrup
- ✔ Brown sugar, malt sugar, inverted sugar, raw sugar, and plain ol' sugar
- ✔ Molasses, honey, and corn sweetener
- ✔ Fruit juice concentrates

High fructose corn syrup (HFCS)

Sucrose — also known as table sugar — is composed of the two sugars glucose and fructose, in roughly equal amounts. Studies suggest that it's broken down and used by our bodies in the same way as when it digests the two sugars, although the jury is still out. One study published in the *Annual Review of Medicine* found that ingesting too much fructose-containing sugars, such as high fructose corn syrup (HFCS) and sucrose, did have a great effect on the risk for heart disease or stroke, due to increased triglycerides and conversion of that excess sugar into fat. However, more research needs to be conducted into whether HFCS really is any different than any excess added sugar.

HFCS makes up about 40 percent of the added sugar in our food supply, because of its low cost relative to other sweeteners. You'll find it in sodas, juices, cereals, salad dressings, nutrition bars — basically anything that is processed for a longer shelf-life.

One thing is for certain. We consume too much added sugar in general — over 130 pounds per person per year. The American Heart Association recommends an upper limit for added sugar at 38 grams per day for men, 25 grams per day for women. That's equivalent to no more than 150 calories and 100 calories per day from added sugar, respectively.

Navigating sugar substitutes

Our food supply is rampant with a variety of sugar substitutes that aren't metabolized the same way as sugar, and therefore, different types of substitutes are used for a variety of reasons:

- ✔ **For weight loss:** They provide fewer calories.
- ✔ **For diabetes:** They have less of an effect on blood sugar levels.
- ✔ **To minimize dental cavities:** They don't stick to the teeth and cause plaque like regular sugar.
- ✔ **To avoid processed foods:** For a more wholesome, natural diet.

Although sugar substitutes can have benefits for the reasons just stated, they also can have a negative effect depending on whether they come from natural or artificial sources.

The lowdown on sugar alcohols

Found in sugar-free chewing gums, candies, frozen desserts, baked goods, and other low-calorie foods, *sugar alcohols* are not really made of sugar or alcohols. They're carbohydrates known as *polyols* whose structure makes them unable to be fully metabolized by the body, and therefore, they contribute fewer calories than other sweeteners. However, they still do contain some calories. How many? The Academy for Nutrition and Dietetics recommends that people using sugar alcohols for blood sugar control to count half the sugar alcohols as carbohydrate. Popular sugar alcohols in foods include xylitol, sorbitol, and mannitol. The Nutrition Facts label includes grams of sugar alcohol in the product.

Part of a sugar alcohol molecule is absorbed and gets converted to energy without need for much insulin. Sounds too good to be true? It kind of is. The other portion of the molecule gets absorbed into the intestine to be fermented by bacteria, which can cause gastrointestinal distress, diarrhea, gas, and bloating. Although sugar alcohols are natural, they're commercially produced and added to products that are typically marketed as healthy, low-calorie, or no sugar added. As far as their safety, in moderation they can be a better option than other sugar substitutes, but keep in mind that these products are not sugar free and when consumed in excess, can affect your blood sugar, not to mention your intestines.

Artificial sweeteners

Although sugar alcohols provide some calories, artificial sweeteners provide essentially none at all. They are not metabolized by any of the normal processes of your metabolism, and they aren't absorbed — but you still get that sweetness when it hits your taste buds. Artificial sweeteners also typically provide much more sweetness per gram than table sugar, so you need to use only a fraction of what you'd use with sugar. However, whenever something sounds too good to be true it probably is.

A study out of the University of Texas found, by looking at the diets of 500 adults, that those who drank diet soda had 70 percent greater increase in their waistlines than non-drinkers close to a decade later. Another study found that for each can of diet soda you drink per day, your risk for obesity increase 41 percent. However, are these people drinking diet soda because they are overweight already and attempting to save calories? It's unclear what's first, the chicken or the egg.

Some additional research found that increased weight with diet sodas could be due to the disconnect between our brains and metabolism. Your taste buds taste sweet, so your body gears up for a load of calories to be delivered, but is confused when it doesn't receive it. Your body releases insulin but arrives at your blood empty-handed with nothing to act upon, leading to cravings. You go out and look for calorie-dense food later on to make up for that and overall eat *more* than you would if you had just chosen regular sugar in the first place. A number of studies have found little or no effect of diet sodas on weight when all factors are taken into account, Therefore, more research needs to be performed, but be aware of artificial sweeteners in your food and in your beverages so you can be mindful of how it affects you, if at all.

There's a lot of buzz surrounding artificial sweeteners and cancer, but in the amounts we typically consume, there's no compelling evidence that risk of cancer is a reason to avoid them. The FDA has established guidelines for acceptable daily intake of these "generally regarded as safe" (GRAS) additives.

Here are the three main artificial sweeteners you'll see on the marketplace and listed in foods:

- ✔ **Aspartame:** Equal, NutraSweet (blue packet)
- ✔ **Saccharin:** Sweet'N Low (pink packet)
- ✔ **Sucralose:** Splenda (yellow packet)

Although it's true that using artificial sweeteners can help keep your caloric intake down in the short term, evidence suggests that you negate those benefits in the long term. Also, food products that contain artificial sweeteners likely contain other additives and preservatives for shelf life stability, taste, and texture. Whenever possible, keep your use of artificial sweeteners to a minimum so that you can be more in tune with your true physical hunger cues.

Natural sweeteners

Natural sweeteners are less refined or processed than artificial sweeteners and are typically made from a plant or fruit. Just because they're natural, though, doesn't make them a healthy option. You'll still get calories and increases in blood sugar and insulin levels with these common natural sugar substitutes:

- ✔ Honey
- ✔ Molasses
- ✔ Maple syrup
- ✔ Agave syrup

Honey does contain antioxidants, and honey and molasses are actually sources of trace minerals like iron, copper, magnesium, and selenium. But don't choose these alternates for those reasons — you can get those minerals and nutrients with true metabolism-boosting foods.

That being said, consuming small amounts of natural sweeteners is better than the processed or artificial stuff. Some research shows that your body breaks it down more seamlessly than a manmade product. But always keep in mind that any sugar in excess of what your body needs gets stored as fat and can slow your metabolic rate.

"Stevia" is an increasingly popular sweetener, sold in packets in grocery stores and coffee shops under various brand names, including Truvia and Pure Via. Stevia is a natural, zero-calorie sweetener processed from the leaves of the South American *Stevia rebaudiana* plant that is 250 times sweeter than sugar. To save calories, stevia is a better addition to your diet than either the artificial or natural-but-still-increases-blood-sugar substitutes. In addition, some studies have found that stevia can actually improve insulin sensitivity and reduce your risk for high blood pressure.

Forgoing solid fats

Growing up, we always had margarine in the refrigerator. We'd learned that butter's saturated fat increased the risk for heart disease, so a slew of margarine products hit the marketplace. These were made with partially *hydrogenated fats*, now commonly known as *trans fats*, which had a hydrogen atom added to an oil molecule so that it became solid like butter.

Partially hydrogenated (trans) fats and solid fats

The food industry loves hydrogenating oils. *Partially* hydrogenating oils makes them more stable and less likely to spoil. They can also withstand heat without breaking down, making them an economical choice for frying foods in commercial fryers. Not only is this ideal for fast food restaurants to make French fries, but it's also ideal for baked goods such as cookies, pastries, pizza dough, and processed snack foods like chips and crackers — not to mention stick margarine.

Margarine was made from heart-healthy fats, so it just had to be healthier than saturated, right? Wrong. Trans fats were deemed to be even more detrimental to heart health than saturated fat from animal products. Both should be avoided as much as possible. In general, solid fats are bad for your health because the more saturated fat a food contains, the more solid it is.

Solid fats include anything that's solid at room temperature, including:

- ✔ Butter
- ✔ Milk fat (the fat in milk is solid — it's just dispersed throughout the liquid using a process called homogenization)
- ✔ Lard (beef or chicken fat)
- ✔ Shortening
- ✔ Stick margarine

And these oils from plant sources are high in saturated or trans fats:

- ✔ Hydrogenated or partially hydrogenated oils
- ✔ Coconut oil
- ✔ Palm and palm kernel oil

Cholesterol, good and bad

Cholesterol is another type of fat which naturally circulates in your blood and is formed by what you eat.

Sources of saturated and trans fats in your diet raise the level of LDL (the "bad") cholesterol in your blood. There are two types of cholesterol:

- ✔ LDL is the "bad" cholesterol that builds up on the inside your arteries and clogs them up, increasing your risk for a heart attack or stroke.
- ✔ HDL is the "good" cholesterol that's actually protective and helps remove LDL from the blood by bringing it to the liver, which gets rid of it.

Why you can go cuckoo for coconut oil

Yes, coconut oil contains high levels of saturated fat, but it doesn't act like typical saturated fats. The majority of oils in our diets are long-chain fatty acids, but coconut oil is a rare source of medium-chain fatty acids (largely lauric acid). The medium chains are more likely to be used for energy instead of being stored in fat cells. Lauric acid, also found in breast milk, has antibacterial, antifungal, and antiviral properties — and increases both HDL and LDL cholesterols but doesn't negatively affect the ratio of the two. That's great because HDL helps balance out the negative effects of LDL cholesterol.

Research has shown that swapping out long-chain fatty acids for medium-chain fatty acids, such as those found in coconut oil, can actually help increase energy expenditure, fat burning, and satiety — and can *decrease* fat storage. In fact, one study found that adding coconut oil to the diet decreased abdominal obesity in women.

Of course, any excess fat in your diet will contribute excess calories, so don't go overboard. And make sure to choose coconut oil that contains no hydrogenated oils to ensure you're reaping the best benefits.

Anything from an animal (meat, dairy, and eggs) contains cholesterol. One large egg contains about 185 milligrams of cholesterol, and eggs get a bad rap for this. However, because our body makes its own cholesterol, the cholesterol you eat doesn't impact your blood cholesterol level as much as we once thought. Saturated fat from foods affects it more, and most of the fat in eggs is unsaturated.

If you do have heart disease, limit your cholesterol intake to 200 milligrams per day and focus on the foods that contain large amounts of saturated or trans fat.

The importance of minimizing trans fats

Trans fats have been shown to negatively impact proper breakdown of glucose and fat in the body, thereby slowing metabolic rate and increasing fat storage. And not only do trans fats increase your LDL (bad) cholesterol, but they *lower* your good cholesterol, HDL. Trans fat also increases inflammation in the body which puts you at risk for chronic diseases like heart disease and diabetes.

Many cities across the country have banned the use of trans fats in restaurants, and in New York City, at least, the effort is paying off. Research over the past five years since the ban took place found that the average trans fats in customers meals has dropped by 2.5 grams, from 3 to 0.5 grams. That's pretty substantial considering that for every 2 percent extra calories from trans fat taken in daily, your risk for heart disease increases by 23 percent. The American Heart Association recommends taking in less than 1 percent of your calories from trans fat.

Even a product with a food label that says "0g Trans Fat" doesn't actually have to be trans fat free. The FDA allows a food that has less than 0.5 grams of trans fat per serving to qualify as "trans fat free." So, even if you're being conscientious about it, you could actually be eating some without knowing it.

Read the ingredient list of your processed snack and baked desserts for "partially hydrogenated oil" to determine whether there is any trace of trans fat in your product.

Cut back on these solid fats and replace them with heart-healthy unsaturated and omega-3 fatty acids (see Chapter 5 for more on these) — instead of refined carbohydrates — to improve your metabolic rate and health.

Table 4-2 lists the top sources of solid fats and the percent each contributes to the U.S. diet. The American Heart Association recommends limiting saturated fats to less than 7 percent of your daily calorie intake. If you're consuming 1,800 calories per day, then 7 percent of your calories = 126. Divide that by 9, because there are 9 calories per gram of fat, and you get a maximum of 14 grams of saturated fat in your diet.

Table 4-2	Top Ten Saturated Fat Sources
Source	*Contribution to Intake (%)*
Full-fat cheese	8.5
Pizza	5.9
Grain desserts (like pies)	5.8
Dairy desserts (like ice cream)	5.6
Chicken dishes	5.5
Sausage, franks, bacon, ribs	4.9
Burgers	4.4
Mexican-based dishes	4.1
Beef dishes	4.1
Reduced-fat milk	3.9

Source: National Cancer Institute, Top Food Sources of Saturated Fat in the U.S. Population, from NHANES 2005–2006

In the late 1990s, when information about how harmful trans fat could really be started surfacing, my mom would still buy margarine. I remember coming home one day and telling her to toss it, but she and my dad had become accustomed to the taste and had believed for so long that it was healthier than butter. The point is that I know it's tough to undo dietary habits. For many years, you may have thought that all fat is unhealthy for you and stuck to all low-fat products (even though many low-fat products on the marketplace add refined sugars for flavor). Now they're telling you there's a fat spectrum of nutritious and not so nutritious fats. Turning knowledge into behavioral change isn't easy.

When it comes to minimizing foods that contain trans fat, take it step by step. For example, if you drink whole milk, next time also buy a carton of skim and try to wean yourself off the whole by pouring a glass half with whole, half with skim. Then slowly increase the proportion of the skim milk in your glass. This is a good analogy for how I want you to view the changes you are making: steady and realistic.

Skipping excess sodium

Sodium chloride, more commonly known as salt, lurks in many of the foods you eat. Sodium functions in the body to regulate nerve impulses, balance fluids, and contract and relax muscles. The typical American diet contains twice the amount of sodium a person needs, and too much sodium puts you at increased risk for high blood pressure and heart disease.

Sodium causes an increase in blood volume, which puts a lot of added burden on your kidneys, which are your filtering system. When that system slows, you are also effectively slowing your metabolic rate.

Dietary Guidelines for Americans, 2010, 7th Edition recommends that you stick to less than 2,300 milligrams of sodium per day — that's one teaspoon of table salt.

The first step is to remove the salt shaker from the table and don't use it while cooking at home. When looking at food labels, go for products that have less than 140 milligrams of sodium per serving. However, almost two-thirds of the sodium we eat comes from food bought in stores, and another fourth comes from food in restaurants. Sodium is also added to many products to preserve shelf-life and flavor.

The sneaky and not-so-sneaky sodium culprits in your diet include the following:

- ✔ Bread (the number one sodium contributor according to the CDC)
- ✔ Cheese
- ✔ Cured, canned, smoked, and processed meats and fish

✔ Canned soups

✔ Salted snack foods like chips, pretzels, popcorn, nuts

✔ Frozen or boxed convenience foods

✔ Fast foods like hamburgers, tacos, pizza, Chinese food

✔ Pickled vegetables like pickles, olives, and relish

✔ Condiments like soy sauce, barbecue sauce, gravy mixes

Anything with salt in its name, such as like garlic salt or onion salt, contains sodium. Products like sea salt offer no benefit and aren't any healthier than regular salt — although they may be marketed as such, they affect your blood pressure and heart health the same way as any other kind. However, you may be able to use less of it, because the crystal size can affect how it tastes and how much of it you use.

Sodium retains water, so the day after you have a big dinner out, you might feel more bloated than normal or gain a couple of pounds on the scale. Don't fret. Just monitor your intake of sodium to help prevent this bloated feeling and keep you feeling your very best.

MSG and your health

MSG, or *monosodium glutamate*, is an amino acid salt flavor enhancer found in many processed, frozen, and soy foods products. It can be in anything from salad dressing to protein powder to soup. There's a theory, with evidence in animal studies only, that MSG can trick taste buds in the same way artificial sweeteners can and cause the pancreas to release more insulin. Also, a study published in the *American Journal of Clinical Nutrition* found that people who eat high amounts of MSG were 33 percent more likely to be overweight by the end of the study. It's just one study, but the author speculates that it's possible MSG could trigger leptin resistance, making it more difficult to sense hunger and satiety. However, more research is needed to make any conclusions.

One thing for sure is that if a product contains MSG, it's likely highly processed. It may also have the potential to trigger migraine headaches. If MSG seems to bother you, avoid it. If not, just focus on keeping your sodium intake down to minimize the processed foods you eat. You can identify food products that can contain MSG by looking for these words in the ingredient list:

✔ Hydrolyzed vegetable protein

✔ Hydrolyzed soy protein

✔ Textured protein

✔ Processed free glutamic acid

✔ Yeast extract

✔ Sodium caseinate

Being aware of BPA

Beyond eating too much of the wrong types of foods and exercising too little, environmental toxins can potentially affect your metabolic rate, too. One toxin that's been well researched over the past decade is Bisphenol A, or BPA. BPA is a synthetic form of estrogen that's in polycarbonate plastic, which is used to manufacture a wide range of products.

BPA is found in the following food-related items:

- ✔ Beverage containers
- ✔ Lining of food and soda cans
- ✔ Plastic plates, bowls, and utensils

Research conducted in rats found that too much BPA altered their hormone and reproductive systems and increased their risk for cancer. One study published in *Environmental Health Perspectives* took fat tissue from humans and found that BPA suppressed a key hormone called adiponectin, which works to increase insulin sensitivity. That suppression could increase risk for diabetes, heart disease, and metabolic syndrome.

According to a study by the CDC, more than 90 percent of Americans have BPA in their urine, and the FDA is supporting efforts to reduce human exposure. BPA has been banned from use in infant feeding bottles in the United States, Canada, and Europe.

More research is definitely needed, but until it's conclusive, here are steps to reduce your exposure:

- ✔ Avoid plastic containers that have a #7 recycling code.
- ✔ Consume fewer canned foods and beverages.
- ✔ Don't microwave plastic containers (it loosens the BPA molecules so they are more likely to leach into your food).
- ✔ Choose a stainless steel or glass water bottle for on-the-go instead of plastic.

Some sober advice on alcohol

Alcohol may help you relax after a long day, but drink too much of it, and your liver will not be happy. Your liver is responsible for breaking down and processing alcohol, and byproducts of this alcohol metabolism can be toxic. Over time, heavy drinkers are at risk for liver diseases like fatty liver, hepatitis, and cirrhosis.

Alcohol offers excess, non-nutritious calories. Also, as with any caloric beverage, your body doesn't register satiety the same way with drinks as with food. As a double whammy, alcohol lowers your inhibitions, and you are more prone to overeating with a few drinks in you.

However, moderate alcohol consumption has some health benefits, such as reducing risk for heart disease and lowering your risk for gallstones. I believe that moderate alcohol intake can be a part of a healthy diet.

Therefore, when drinking, do so in moderation. The *Dietary Guidelines for Americans, 2010*, 7th Edition recommends one drink per day for women and two for men. One drink = 12 ounces of beer = 5 ounces of wine = 1.5 ounces 80 proof distilled spirits.

Be mindful of the amount of calories you consume through booze. Anything made with a drink mix, fruit juice, or soda can rack 'em up. For example, a 6-ounce margarita contains 300 calories and 58 grams of sugar — which can get converted to fat in your body.

Use these tips to keep your calories down when drinking:

- ✔ Choose wine or light beer.
- ✔ Dilute your drink with sparkling water.
- ✔ Alternate alcohol drinks with non-alcoholic drinks like water to keep calories down and prevent getting too tipsy.
- ✔ Order a spirit on the rocks.
- ✔ Ditch pre-made mixers that have added and artificial sugars.
- ✔ When using fruit juice as a mixer, choose 100 percent juice and keep it under 6 ounces.

Whenever you're drinking, eat something first. Don't go into it on an empty stomach. Have a game plan so you're more likely to make that healthy food decision you planned before the night. As the saying goes, "Failing to plan is planning to fail."

Identifying What Has Thwarted Your Efforts

It's time to take out the magnifying glass to examine your eating behaviors. By identifying where you can benefit from improvements, you can then pinpoint the behaviors you need to improve upon when it comes to your diet and lifestyle.

Clients come into me all the time and say, "I eat very healthy, so I'm not sure why I'm not losing weight." By being mindful and holding yourself account-able for everything you put into your body, you will recognize that you are eating more than you think or too many of the metabolism-busting foods that you need to minimize. But even when you take a closer look, you can ignore reality or sabotage yourself from achieving the results you want.

Keeping a food diary

If you ask me, "What's the one thing that has worked for most of your clients to improve their diet?" the answer is simply keeping a food diary.

Many are turned off by the idea. They don't want to be bothered to take the time to monitor everything that goes into their mouths. But maybe this will make you change your tune: Keeping a food diary has been shown to be the most powerful predictor of weight loss. In one study published in the *American Journal of Preventive Medicine*, those who kept a diary six days per week lost about twice as much as those who kept the diary only one day a week or not at all.

The food diary effect is two pronged. First, it keeps you accountable for what you're eating and drinking. This can be a motivator to not to eat those candies on your coworker's desk or take cheese samples at the supermarket. Second, you get a feel for the amounts you are eating and can identify correlations between food, mood, cravings, and your weight. For example, maybe you were feeling very light-headed in the afternoon, and upon review of your food diary, you noticed your lunch wasn't all that substantial.

A general food diary I have my clients keep has headings like this:

Time	*Food/Beverage*	*Portion Size*	*Hunger Scale*	*Mood*

But even if you just keep the food/beverage column and don't focus on any-thing else, it's a good start. Timing helps you understand how long you go between meals. Timing can affect your metabolism and mood — in addition to affecting the types of foods, beverages, and combinations you're consuming.

Rating your hunger on a scale from 1–10 can help you become more in tune with physical hunger cues. If 0 is starving and 10 is uncomfortably full, you should eat when you are at a 2–3 and stop at a 7–8.

As for mood, include a note about how you feel at the time of your meal. This helps you be more mindful of whether you're eating because you're hungry, stressed, tired, or experiencing other emotions.

Plating portions

Although increasing portion size isn't the sole cause for expanding waistlines and sluggish metabolisms, Americans suffer from portion distortion. An abundance of inexpensive foods is available in large quantities in our food supply. For one example, a bagel 20 years ago was 3 inches in diameter and 140 calories. Nowadays you'd be hard pressed to find one smaller than 5–6 inches, at double the calories.

Even if you're making nutritious choices with foods, big portions could be sabotaging your best efforts.

When it comes to portioning your food, start by focusing on achieving a balance of nutrients at each meal. In 2011, the USDA released MyPlate (Figure 4-2) to replace the decades-old Food Guide Pyramid.

Figure 4-2:
MyPlate
helps you
picture how
to balance
food groups
on your
plate.

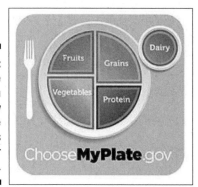

Image courtesy of USDA

Although you don't need to eat all the food groups shown in Figure 4-2 at every meal, you do need to have a balance of heart-healthy fats, high-fiber carbs, and lean protein at every meal to keep your metabolism moving and your energy levels high.

The Academy for Nutrition and Dietetics Exchange Lists (shown in Table 4-3) is a good place to get started on monitoring your serving sizes.

Table 4-3	General Serving Sizes of Food Groups	
Food Group	*Serving Size*	*Approximate Calories/ Serving*
Vegetables	1 cup raw or ½ cup cooked	25
Fruits	1 small apple, banana, orange	60
	½ grapefruit or mango	
	1 cup berries	
	¼ cup dried fruit	
Fat free milk	1 cup milk	90
	¾ cup yogurt	
Very lean protein	1 ounce poultry without skin and fish	35
	½ cup beans	
Lean protein	1 ounce dark meat poultry without skin	55
	Leaf beef, pork tenderloin, ham	
	¼ cup low fat cottage cheese	
Starches	1 slice whole wheat bread	80
	1 ounce bagel	
	½ cup pasta, rice, potato	
Fats	1 teaspoon oil	45
	⅛ avocado	

Based on the Academy for Nutrition and Dietetics Exchange List

The exact amount you need at each meal depends on your calorie level. So, if you are aiming for 1,500 calories per day, to spread your calorie intake out evenly you want to have about 400–500 calories per meal and 200–300 for a snack. (I expand on ideal composition of those meals in Chapter 5 and talk more about how to eyeball portions on the fly and make the best decisions when dining out in Chapter 14.)

Instituting an actionable plan

You may have tried and stopped trying to make healthy changes in the past. Let me ask you this: How much planning did you really do beforehand? Were you just following someone else's advice or dieting blindly? Or were you truly setting and achieving realistic goals that you set for yourself? In this section, I highlight the three parts of starting and sticking to healthy habits for the long term.

Setting realistic goals

Goal setting helps you stay motivated in the long term and short term. You can set goals for any aspect of your life: your diet, exercise, personal issues, or career trajectory if you feel like you've been unable to stay motivated or you have no willpower to make changes. By setting attainable goals, you can stay on a path to transforming your wishes into reality.

On the first page of your food diary notebook, write down your ultimate or "big picture" goal. Writing goals down makes them real and visual. You can refer to your list when you've lost sight of why you're trying to make healthy changes. Also, goals help you realize and remember where your priorities lie.

Some examples of big picture goals might include the following:

- ✔ I want to maximize my metabolic rate for improved energy
- ✔ I want to be within a healthy weight range for my height
- ✔ I want to eat more nutritiously to reduce my risk for disease
- ✔ I want to run a marathon next year

Once you have your big picture goal, each week set smaller, daily tasks that you can focus on as you work toward the ultimate goal, such as starting to eat breakfast, adding more fruits and vegetables, cutting out soda, going for walks — whatever habit is realistic and sustainable for you. Achieving those small tasks helps you build self-confidence and motivation to keep going.

You might have a number in mind — a magic number of pounds, at which point you think you'll be happy with your weight, or the number of pounds you want to lose, or a pace you want to run, or how many times per week you will make time for exercise. Then, if you don't achieve it, you feel like a failure and give up. Your goal should be performance based, not outcome based. You're not as likely to succeed if you say, "I want to weigh X amount of pounds" as you are if you say, "I will cut out 500 calories per day and here are the swaps I will make." Be positive and kind to yourself, and you will be much more likely to succeed.

Planning healthy rewards

If you've decided to treat yourself to an extra serving of ice cream (or any other favorite, fun, or decadent food) as a reward for being extra diligent about what you're eating, you're not alone. I'm certainly not against the occasional splurge here and there. But the reason for a splurge shouldn't be because of recent healthy eating behaviors.

Psychologically, rewarding yourself with food can make you idealize foods as only able to be consumed when you're "good," and can further perpetuate the detrimental good/bad mentality discussed earlier in this chapter. Rewarding yourself with food makes you more prone to get caught up in emotional eating or ignore your physical hunger cues and eat because you "deserve it."

Instead, plan rewards for reaching your short and long term goals that *don't* have to do with food. Plan rewards and focus on self-care or improved well-ness in other areas. Here are some ideas:

- ✔ Treat yourself to a manicure or give yourself one.
- ✔ Get a spa treatment.
- ✔ Go to a sporting event or set aside time to play a sport with friends.
- ✔ Visit a local museum, theater, or art gallery.
- ✔ Take a relaxing bath with scented oils.
- ✔ Take a class with a friend (exercise, photography, arts and crafts, you name it).
- ✔ Put money in a jar towards that new technology gadget you've been eyeing.
- ✔ Go to a department store for a free makeover at a makeup counter.

Whatever you do, make sure it's something you wouldn't do normally and that makes you feel good inside and out.

Tracking your progress

In the past, you've used the scale to track your progress, but it's important to start thinking beyond weight. When the scale doesn't go down, you could think you're not being successful, but remember your success is measured by more than your weight. It's measured by reaching those smaller tasks and goals, having more energy, improving your blood levels of cholesterol and sugar when you're tested at the doctor, and enhancing your self-confidence and feelings of self-worth.

With a to-do list, you place a big checkmark next to a completed task — do so when you achieve your goals for the day, week, or month. You can use an online tool to keep this list, track your food, activity, how you feel, and weight goals. I work for one so I'm biased towards CalorieCount.com, but there are plenty of others online. These are also available as mobile apps, to help you keep track on the go:

- ✔ www.CalorieCount.com
- ✔ www.SparkPeople.com
- ✔ www.Fitbit.com (tied in with a pedometer and calorie burn tracker)

Keeping an eye on all these aspects of your progress is another way to be mindful and stay motivated to stay on a healthy track toward improved health.

For more details and help on changing your ways, see my free article "Taking Care to Change Your Lifestyle" at www.dummies.com/URL.

Chapter 5

Choosing Metabolism-Boosting Foods and Nutrients

In This Chapter

▶ Figuring out the what and why of the best foods for your metabolism

▶ Understanding the key nutrients and when you need to take a supplement

▶ Discovering the spices that boost your rate (and add flavor)

▶ Understanding when to choose organic foods

*I*f your body is like a car, then your metabolism is the engine churning away to make sure you're up and running. You only have one body, and it requires premium fuel to work as best it can. If you're feeding it anything else, it can operate, but needs to work harder — too hard — to process this inefficient fuel. In other words, you're more likely to burn out quickly and live with a sluggish metabolism.

This chapter explains what makes up this premium fuel and how it helps you function at your best. Focus on adding these foods and nutrients to your diet so that you aren't deprived and are motivated to continue doing so because you'll feel better, have more energy, and begin to realize that boosting your metabolism doesn't have to be so hard after all. The best food for you can also taste good, and adding spices and herbs can make it all the more enjoyable — plus they can also add a little boost.

This chapter also answers some burning (pun intended) questions that I often hear from clients, such as when to take a supplement, which are the best ones for your metabolic rate, and whether to buy organic foods.

Metabolism-Boosting Foods and Nutrients

Whether or not you start removing the metabolism busters discussed in Chapter 4 from your diet, you can start adding in metabolism-*boosting* foods and nutrients. Part of the beauty of these foods is that not only are they the top premium fuels you can find, but they also help keep you more satisfied and leave little room for your less-than-nutritious options. Because they're real and found in nature (with some tweaks), they work your metabolism engine in the best way.

Understanding how these foods improve your metabolic rate helps you keep your eye on the prize. Maybe you never knew the nitty-gritty before, or maybe you just need a reminder. Either way, knowledge is power when it comes to making nutritious choices, and I provide tips on how everyone can start chowing down on these boosters stat.

Whole grains and fiber

Your body thrives on getting carbohydrates to use as energy. When you don't get enough of those, your body needs to break down protein to use instead, which puts unnecessary pressure on your body. You need that protein for other functions, such as hair and nail growth and building and maintaining muscle tissue. So, getting enough carbs is important. But taking it a step further, choosing whole grains over refined grains is key to keeping your energy high and your metabolism strong. Make sure at least half your grains are whole grains, which means at minimum three servings per day.

In general, 1 serving of grain = 1 slice of bread = ½ cup cooked cereal = 1 cup cold, ready-to-eat cereal. These values are derived from the Academy for Nutrition and Dietetics' Exchange List, which was created with people with diabetes in mind to monitor their carbohydrate serving sizes. Although serving sizes will vary, read a food label to discover your grain serving — which should contain 80 calories and 15 grams of carbohydrate. Or for a visual, if you're looking at your plate, grains should take up about a fourth of the real estate.

Refined carbohydrates — ones that are processed and stripped of their natural nutrition — can be used for energy also, but cause a rapid increase and decrease in your blood sugar levels, which leaves you feeling irritable, fatigued, and hungry.

Many of the metabolism-boosting foods are full of fabulous fiber. Fiber helps stoke your metabolism and maintain a healthy weight because it fills you up on fewer calories than refined foods do. Not to mention it's also beneficial for heart health, helps lower cholesterol, and works to prevent certain cancers. Fiber literally grabs toxins and drags them out of your body — a natural "detox," if you will.

There are two main types of dietary fiber. They have different functions, but both are important to your health. One's not better for you than the other; in general, you just want to get a mix of both in your diet:

- **Soluble fiber:** *Soluble* means it latches onto water and forms a gel, which slows movement of food through your digestive tract. This is great for stabilizing your blood sugar levels. These soluble fibers also interfere with the absorption of bad LDL cholesterol, keeping your level of that lower. That's why, when you need to lower their cholesterol, your doctor might tell you to start by eating oatmeal in the morning. But soluble fiber is actually found in all fruits, some veggies, nuts, and seeds, too. You can also get it in the form of psyllium (a fiber found in some foods and fiber supplements).

- **Insoluble fiber**: Insoluble fiber doesn't dissolve in water. It provides bulk and helps prevent constipation by speeding up the passing of food and waste through your digestive tract. Insoluble fiber is mainly found in vegetables, some fruits, seeds, nuts, and whole grains.

The average American only gets about 15 grams of fiber in their diet, but really needs at least 25–30 grams per day.

Choosing more whole grains, as well as the other metabolism boosters like fruits, veggies, nuts, seeds, and beans, is an important way to meet those needs and keeps your digestive system functioning the best it can. Fiber helps keep your blood sugar levels stable and keeps you feeling fuller for longer.

A slew of products on the marketplace add fiber — to yogurts, beverages, and even candy bars. But these products are not as good for you as the real thing. Therefore, be wary of fiber claims on packages and read the ingredient label to see if it contains a naturally occurring whole grain or additive form of fiber such as inulin. A product with inulin isn't bad for you, but whenever possible, go for the real whole grain.

The 2010 Dietary Guidelines for Americans recommends making half your grains whole — but the more, the better in general, of course. Having refined grains or white breads for one serving per day is fine in moderation, as long as you pair it with other foods such as green leafy veggies, lean protein, and heart-healthy fats that slow the absorption of glucose into your bloodstream.

Whole grains go beyond whole wheat breads, whole-grain pasta, and brown rice. Expand your grain horizons with these foods:

✔ Barley

✔ Buckwheat

✔ Bulgur

✔ Whole-grain corn or corn meal

✔ Farro

✔ Freekeh

✔ Millet

✔ Oats or oatmeal

✔ Quinoa

✔ Rice (brown and wild)

✔ Whole rye

✔ Sorghum

✔ Spelt

✔ Popcorn

✔ Wheatberries

✔ Whole-wheat flour

In order for a food product to really, truly qualify as a whole grain, 100 percent of the kernel — including the bran and endosperm — must be present. The nutrients found in whole grains, such as fiber, magnesium, and zinc, have been researched for their benefits on metabolism (more on that later in this chapter).

Unfortunately, only about 10–15 percent of the products on the shelf in your supermarket are whole grain. So how are you supposed to make sure you are getting enough of it? You need to make sure the product lists the word *whole* before the word *grain* in the first position of the ingredient list.

The closer an ingredient is to the top of the ingredient list, the more weight it contains in the product. Choose breads whose packages boast *100% whole grain* — but skip all other claims, like *made with whole grain* or *multigrain*.

Try these swaps to boost your whole grain intake:

✔ Swap out corn flakes for breakfast, and swap in steel cut oats. Get creative with toppings. I like to add peanut butter. Other favorites include flaxseed, dried or fresh fruit, and cinnamon.

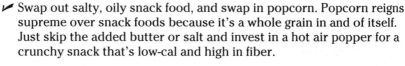

✔ Swap out salty, oily snack food, and swap in popcorn. Popcorn reigns supreme over snack foods because it's a whole grain in and of itself. Just skip the added butter or salt and invest in a hot air popper for a crunchy snack that's low-cal and high in fiber.

I advise limiting microwave popcorn. The lining of the bags contains a chemical coating that can be broken down into a carcinogen, and the popcorn itself is primed with an FDA-approved chemical called diacetyl that has been shown to cause lung disease in popcorn factory workers. That's because they're around it 24/7, so if you have a bag of microwave popcorn once in a while, you'll probably be ok.

✔ Swap out white bread products, and swap in whole grain breads, cereals, bagels, crackers, even waffles. When baking, try mixing in half whole wheat flour and half white flour.

✔ Swap in whole grain bread crumbs or oats to add texture to ground beef and turkey patties.

✔ Swap in whole grain breads when making French toast, whole wheat pitas for mini pizzas, whole wheat tortillas for Mexican night, brown rice in chili, and buckwheat noodles in Asian stir-fries.

✔ Experiment with grains like quinoa or barley as a side at dinner instead of your staples. Check out Chapter 9 for creative ideas. If that's too adventurous for you, go with whole grain pastas and brown rice for the upgrade.

As you're adding more whole grains and fiber to your diet, make sure you're drinking plenty of water. Otherwise, the added bulk could leave you bloated and constipated. Because your body is made of up to 60 percent water, drinking it helps prevent you from feeling dehydrated and keeps your energy levels high. (See Chapter 2 for tips on how to meet your water needs and when to know you're having enough.)

Eating from the rainbow

Do you wish I was talking about that popular brand of rainbow-colored sugary candies? Well, I'm not. But just as each color represents a different flavor in the candy, each pigment present in fruits and vegetables is due to a compound that serves up different health benefits. Fruits and veggies provide a more natural sweet fix that's loaded with fiber, vitamins, minerals, and other metabolism-maximizing goodies.

If you aren't the biggest fruit and veggie fan, and you think "If only I liked fruits and veggies I could lose weight and feel great," you aren't alone. Clients come to me with this mentality. The good news is they leave with new ways of enjoying fruits and vegetables of all colors.

TIP

Aim for 4–5 servings each fruit and vegetable per day:

✔ **Fruits:** 1 serving = ½ cup fresh fruit = ½ cup juice = ¼ dried fruit. (A serving contains 60 calories and 15 grams of carbohydrate.)

✔ **Vegetables:** 1 serving = ½ cup cooked = 1 cup raw leafy vegetable. (A serving contains 25 calories and 5 grams of carbohydrate.)

Check out the nutrients of the color spectrum shown in Table 5-1 and pick out at least one or two options per color to incorporate into your diet. For each, I list the main phytonutrient (the main compound that gives the plant its color). But each group contains numerous vitamins and minerals, many of which act as antioxidants. *Antioxidants* protect your body from damage from free radicals, improve heart health, and according to research can help boost sugar and fat metabolism. The more you add from each color, the better variety you'll get.

Table 5-1	Color Spectrum Fruits and Vegetables		
Color	*Fruits/Vegetables*	*Power Nutrient*	*Nutrient Function*
Red	Red apple, beets, cherries, cranberries, pink/red grapefruit, pomegranate, raspberries, strawberries, tomato	Lycopene	May reduce risk for cancer
Orange/ Yellow	Apricot, butternut squash, cantaloupe, carrots, orange, papaya, peach, persimmons, pineapple, pumpkin, sweet corn, sweet potato, tangerine	Beta-carotene	Converted to vitamin A for eye health and immunity
Green	Artichoke, asparagus, avocado, leafy green veggies, broccoli, Brussels sprouts, celery, cucumbers, collards, honeydew, kale, spinach, zucchini	Chlorophyll	These are chock-full of vitamins and minerals that protect against disease
Blue/ Purple	Blackberries, blueberries, eggplant, figs, grapes, plums	Anthocyanins	Antioxidants like resveratrol protect cells from damage and improve memory function
White	Banana, cauliflower, garlic, ginger, jicama, mushrooms, onions, potato	Anthoxanthins	Allicin can serve to lower cholesterol and blood pressure

Adding more fruits and vegetables to your day can help you get more bang for your buck. In other words, you can fill up on fewer calories, satisfied, and have more energy due to the fiber and vitamins you're getting. Fruits and vegetables have a high water content, meaning you take in more volume than you do with denser, nutritionally poor food. Table 5-2 outlines an example of adding color to your meals and how the nutrition tallies up.

Table 5-2	Adding Color (and Volume) to Your Plate	
Meal	*Dreary Day*	*Colorful Day*
Breakfast	2 waffles, 1 tablespoon syrup	2 waffles with 1 cup of berries
Lunch	Turkey (3 ounces), 2 slices whole wheat bread, 1 ounce chips	Turkey (3 ounces) with lettuce, tomato, 2 slices whole wheat bread, 20 baby carrots, apple with 1 tablespoon peanut butter
Snack	6 ounces yogurt, 2 graham crackers	6 ounces yogurt, 3 slices dried mango
Dinner	2 slices pizza, 2 garlic knots	2 slices veggie pizza with whole wheat crust, spinach salad with 1 tablespoon olive oil
Dessert	Chocolate pudding	Chocolate pudding with 1 cup skim milk
Total Nutrition	1,400 calories, 10 grams fiber, Below needs for vitamins A, C, calcium.	1,400 calories, 30 grams fiber, Meets RDA for vitamins A, C, calcium.

Making room for fruits and vegetables doesn't have to break the bank. Here are ideas of how you can add color on a budget:

- ✔ **Go frozen.** Frozen fruits and vegetables are less expensive and not as perishable as fresh. They are frozen at peak of ripeness as well, which means they're likely to retain *more* nutrition than fresh foods that lose nutrients during traveling and handling.

- ✔ **Go in season.** When fruits and vegetables are in season, they're less expensive. This is another reason why frozen produce is cool, too — you can buy out of season for cheap.

- ✔ **Go local.** Fruits and veggies are cheaper at your local street or farmer's market. At your supermarket, look for deals in the circular, which is typically located as you enter the store.

- ✔ **Forgo prepackaged and precut.** Although perhaps more convenient, on top of the cost of the fruit, you're paying for the labor and materials that go into cutting and packaging these products. If you're not buying frozen, buy whole fruits and vegetables and do the slicing and dicing yourself.

To juice or not to juice?

Juicing fruits and vegetables is very popular right now — both at home, on-the-go, and via bottles in health food stores around the country. The bad news is that the process of juicing removes fiber because the skin and pulp of the fruit is left out. Also, you don't get the same amount of nutrition because many of the nutrients are concentrated in the skin. While more sophisticated juicers can keep the skin and pulp, with any food, you have to be aware of calorie content. And even though fiber is still present, juicing breaks it down, so you don't get the same benefit from bulk.

Adding multiple servings of fruit to one 8 ounce glass can add up fast. The problem with these calories from beverages is that your body doesn't recognize them the same way as if you ate the food whole. The process of chewing tastes longer than drinking, and you're more likely to be satisfied for longer if you eat the components whole instead of blended or juiced.

All that being said, I'm not a complete juice hater. But there's a time, a place, and a best practice:

- ✔ If you're one of those people who doesn't like fruits and veggies or has a lot of difficulty making room for the 4–5 servings of each per day, juicing can be a good option to get some antioxidants and nutrients in.

- ✔ Make sure you add a lean protein and/or heart-healthy fat to the mix so that it can be a meal or snack and satisfy you longer. For substance, add nut butter, low-fat milk or yogurt, avocado, or seeds such as chia or flax.

- ✔ If drinking market-bought juice, stick to 100 percent fruit juice at a ½ cup serving.

When *not* to juice: Don't fast with juices as an extreme weight-loss tool. It won't last for the long term, and you'll be depriving your body of essential nutrients — therefore slowing your metabolic rate.

Incorporating low-fat dairy

As a kid, you drank milk for strong bones. As an adult, you can choose low-fat dairy products to burn more fat (and also maintain bones and reduce blood pressure). A study published in *Nutrition and Metabolism* found that people who drank the recommended amount of dairy — about 3–4 servings per day— were more likely to have increased metabolic rates and greater fat oxidation during weight maintenance. The subjects were also able to take in more calories than the low-dairy group without weight regain.

But that doesn't mean that you can guzzle a gallon of milk with your fast-food hamburger to counteract its effects.

Adding dairy to an otherwise healthful diet will have the best impact on your metabolic rate. Have a low-fat yogurt with breakfast, add a cup of skim milk to your snack, and add part-skim cheese to your dinner to get your servings in with ease.

Calcium plays a role in fat storage. Getting the recommended amount of calcium can equate to burning 100 more calories per day at rest! That adds up to a weight loss of over 10 pounds per year. It also means less fat storage, especially when the calcium is consumed in the form of low-fat dairy. In a study out of the University of Tennessee, women who consumed 3 cups of low-fat yogurt per day lost 60 percent more body fat than those who didn't.

Calcium is found in non-dairy forms, either naturally or fortified, and those can help you meet your needs too. Aim for about 1,200 milligrams of calcium per day. If you aren't able to meet those needs through diet (have a look at Table 5-3), a supplement can help — but my motto is *food first whenever possible*. Also, as you'll see in Table 5-3, when a product is low-fat, the calcium content is typically greater than a full fat product — bonus!

Table 5-3	Calcium Sources	
Food	*Serving Size*	*Calcium per serving (mg)*
Yogurt, plain, low-fat	8 ounces	415
Orange juice, calcium-fortified	6 ounces	375
Mozzarella, part-skim	1.5 ounces	333
Sardines, canned in oil, with bones	3 ounces	325
Milk, nonfat	8 ounces	299
Milk, whole	8 ounces	276
Tofu, firm, made with calcium sulfate	½ cup	253
Salmon, pink, canned, w. bones	3 ounces	181
Instant breakfast drinks, powder w water	8 ounces	105–250
Frozen yogurt, vanilla, soft serve	½ cup	103
Ready-to-eat cereal, calcium-fortified	1 cup	100–1,000
Kale, fresh, cooked	1 cup	94
Soy beverage, calcium fortified	8 ounces	80-500

Source: USDA Nutrient Database

Another benefit of choosing low-fat yogurt and cheeses are the probiotics that lie within. *Probiotics* are live organisms like bacteria and yeast that help keep our guts healthy. Many digestive disorders result from problems with the natural bacteria found in the lining of our intestines. Probiotics can help reduce inflammation and keep your digestive system healthy and strong. The FDA doesn't regulate probiotics (yet), so when looking at products, look for the strains *Lactobacillus* and *Bifidobacteria*, and choose reputable brands. Also make sure the label specifies "live" or "active" cultures. You may also want to check out the excellent reference book *Probiotics For Dummies* (Wiley, 2012).

Pros of protein

Most Americans get enough protein. Okay, we get double the protein we need. For the average joe, that's okay as long as that protein is from lean sources — meaning low in artery-clogging saturated fat — and as long as what you're consuming isn't exceeding the amount of calories you need. But if you're on a restricted or vegetarian diet, or just aren't eating enough, you may need to focus on adding the right kinds of protein back into your diet.

We need protein to build and maintain tissues in our bodies. We have protein in all our cells, which is regularly broken down and replaced by what we get in our diet. Amino acids are the building blocks of protein, and our bodies can't make them on their own, which is why they are called *essential* amino acids: we must get them from our diet.

There are two main types of protein sources based on their amino acid content:

- ✔ **Complete proteins:** These contain all the essential amino acids we need and are animal based (because those animals need the same amino acids that we do). Complete proteins are found in meat, fish, poultry, dairy, and eggs.

- ✔ **Incomplete proteins:** These do not contain one or more of the amino acids but still offer up a source of protein. This includes plant sources like beans, grains, nuts, and seeds. It used to be thought that you needed to eat combinations of these foods together at the same meal to create the complete protein from the complementary proteins, for example rice and beans together provide all the essential amino acids. But now it's accepted that as long as you consume the foods within the same day, you will get the nutrients you need.

No matter where it's coming from, getting about 4 ounces of protein per meal has advantages for your metabolic rate and ability to lose weight. A study published in the *American Journal of Clinical Nutrition* found that, per calorie ingested, more weight loss occurs with a high-protein diet versus high-carbohydrate diet. Some possible reasons for this include the following:

- ✔ Protein helps build and maintain muscle mass, which then burns more at rest.

- ✔ Excess carbohydrate calories are more readily changed into and stored as fat.

- ✔ It takes longer to metabolize protein, so you feel more satisfied, resulting in decreased hunger.

Choose leaner sources of protein to save on calories and saturated fat that you might be consuming with fatty meats and full-fat dairy. Also consider including plant-based sources of protein in your diet. Try the following swaps:

✔ Forgo the rib-eye or T-bone steak and go with sirloin, top round, tenderloin, and bottom round cuts — and trim visible fat.

✔ Go with white meat over dark when it comes to poultry and remove the skin to save on saturated fat calories.

✔ Don't forget about preparation. Choose grilled, broiled, or baked lean meats and fish instead of fried or sautéed.

✔ Add beans or tofu instead of meat to soups, chili, salads, and pastas.

✔ Pick low-fat dairy products like skim or 1 percent milk, part-skim cheese, low-fat yogurts — including high-protein Greek yogurt for a lean-protein, calcium boost.

✔ Get a serving of nuts or nut butter with your snack to keep your energy level high for hours between meals.

✔ If you're a carnivore or herbivore, you can benefit from the protein found in whole grains, specifically quinoa.

Do you need protein powder?

Protein powders are a popular nutritional supplement, not just with muscle men at the gym but sold in any smoothie joint or as premade mixes in the grocery store. They are typically made of whey, casein, and soy proteins. But do you really need protein powder to meet your nutrition needs? It can be helpful in some cases such as if you're recovering from surgery and need more protein for wound healing, or you're starting to eat vegan and haven't yet figured out how to meet your needs through diet.

On average, you need about 0.8–1.0 grams of protein per kilogram of body weight per day. Athletes can require up to 1.8 grams per kilogram maximum. So, if you're 150 pounds (divided by 2.2 for kilograms = 68 kilograms) and

moderately exercise, you really only need 55–70 grams of protein per day, and potentially up to 125 grams maximum of you do intense strength training. It might sounds like a lot, but if you had 8 ounces of meat throughout the day you'd get about 56 grams just from that, not including any other sources of high biological or trace proteins from grains and produce.

If you aren't meeting your nutrient needs, protein powder might be a good way to get it in, but otherwise there's no benefit from doing so if you have a normal, healthy diet. There also isn't much convincing research that choosing whey, casein, or soy can help build muscle better than another type.

The power of omega-3 fatty acids

It seems like every day there is a new health benefit that omega-3 fatty acids bestow upon us: they're good for your heart, improve arthritis, reduce depression, help with hot flashes during menopause, and now they help boost your metabolism?

But what are omega-3 fatty acids, where can you find them, and why are they all the rage?

Just as amino acids of protein are *essential* — meaning we need to get them from our diet — so are omega-3 fatty acids. Our bodies cannot make these fats, but they're required for many functions such as building cell membranes and controlling blood clotting and inflammation in the body.

Most Americans don't get enough omega-3 fatty acids. There are three kinds found in foods:

- Eicosapentaenoic acid (EPA) and docosahexaenoic acid (DHA) are mostly found in fatty fish like salmon and tuna. These're easiest for your body to use.

- Alpha-linolenic acid (ALA) is found in nuts such as walnuts, seeds and seed products such as flaxseed and flax oil, vegetable oils such as soybean and canola oil, green leafy vegetables such as Brussels sprouts and kale, and in some grass-fed animal products. It's also often used to fortify products like eggs, peanut butter, and granola bars. It's more difficult for your body to use this type of omega-3.

Aim to get at least one rich source of omega-3 into your diet every day:

- Eat two servings of fatty fish per week, such as tuna, wild salmon, and sardines.

- Add ground flaxseed (flaxmeal) or walnuts to oatmeal, salads, and yogurts.

- Choose olive, canola, and soybean oil for salad dressings instead of creamy ranch or Caesar.

- Scramble up omega-3 fortified eggs in the morning (or for dinner!).

If you aren't able to get omega-3s into your diet, you might consider taking a supplement.

But check with your doctor before taking omega-3 supplements, such as fish oil which functions as a blood thinner — in high doses, or when taken with other meds, it could have a negative effect on your health.

Saturated and trans fat in your diet can negate the positive effects of omega-3, so make sure you keep those to a minimum (see Chapter 4 for how to do that). Instead, opt for omega-3s and other sources of unsaturated fats, like avocado, nuts, nut butter, and seeds.

So how do omega-3s affect metabolism? Getting enough fat is important for satiety — you feel fuller longer when you get a serving of fat in your meal. There's evidence that omega-3s have an even better effect than other fats due to stimulation of *leptin*, the hormone that tells your brain you are full. A study published in *Appetite* found that people who were overweight and fed more omega-3s felt less hunger while losing weight.

When there's not enough leptin circulating in your body, there's a higher level of the neurotransmitter neuropeptide Y, which signals the hunger reflex. An increase in neuropeptide Y can decrease thyroid function and your metabolic rate.

What else can omega-3s do for you?

- ✔ Reduce symptoms of arthritis like stiffness and joint pain.

- ✔ Lower risk for depression; fish oil may boost the effects of antidepressants.

- ✔ Improve visual and neurological development of infants in utero.

- ✔ May lower triglycerides and reduce risk for heart disease (although emerging research contradicts this).

- ✔ Preliminary research shows it could reduce your risk for Alzheimer's disease and dementia.

Although getting more fatty fish is a great idea to boost your health, you want to choose wisely. Some fish have higher levels of environmental toxins like mercury, which comes from industrial pollution. Fish absorb the mercury that's released into the water, and it builds up inside them. Bigger fish and those that are farm raised have higher toxin levels. Women of child-bearing age, pregnant women, and children should heed the following guidelines:

- ✔ Avoid fish that are high in mercury: shark, swordfish, tilefish, king mackerel. Limit farmed fish.

- ✔ Choose these lower-in-mercury options: canned light tuna, wild salmon, shrimp, Pollock, and catfish — up to 12 ounces per week.

✔ If consuming fish caught by friends or family in local waters, but you're unable to find information about the mercury content, stick to less than 6 ounces and don't consume any other fish that week.

You can also refer to the Environmental Protection Agency's website at www.epa.gov for more information about the fish around where you live.

Nuts, seeds, and beans galore

Whether or not you're vegetarian, nuts, seeds, and beans are nutrition powerhouses that help keep your metabolism moving efficiently. They all contain lean protein and fiber; nuts and seeds contain heart-healthy fats that keep you feeling satisfied and energized.

This section lists my top picks and the nutrients they contain.

Nuts over these nuts

✔ **Almonds:** These are rich in vitamin E, a powerful antioxidant that protects heart health, and magnesium, a mineral that's important to metabolism. The fiber content and unique texture of almonds improve satiety, and in 2012, the USDA discovered that almonds may provide 20 percent fewer calories than scientists previously believed.

Make your own trail mix including almonds, dried fruit, and even a sprinkle of dark chocolate chips for a sweet, satisfying snack. One serving (1 ounce) = 24 kernels.

✔ **Brazil nuts:** These are a great source of selenium, a mineral that has been researched to improve fat metabolism. Nosh on them whole and mixed in with popcorn for a filling and energizing snack. But limit yourself to two kernels per day. Too much selenium can be toxic, and two per day is plenty.

✔ **Pistachios:** Pistachios contain B vitamins, specifically B6, which help with energy metabolism. I like them because 1 ounce gives you 47 kernels, so your mouth stays busy longer. Eat them straight up (be even more satisfied by taking the time to de-shell) or mix in with salads or pasta dishes.

✔ **Walnuts:** These are the best nut source of omega-3 fatty acids, which improve satiety and have been shown to help with cognitive function. Add chopped walnuts to your morning oatmeal to balance out the meal and help you stay full until lunchtime. One serving = 14 halves.

Super seeds

✔ **Chia seeds:** Yes, these are the seeds you spread over your Chia Pet to make sprouted hair grow. Who knew they were nutrition powerhouses? Chia seeds contain omega-3 and a balance of soluble and insoluble fiber to help keep your blood sugar steady and make your digestion work more to keep your metabolism moving. Add a tablespoon to your yogurt or salad, blend with smoothies, and add to baked goods.

✔ **Flaxseeds** contain heart-healthy fats, fiber, and lignans, which are powerful antioxidants that may protect against breast and other types of cancer. You need to grind them to release their nutrient power or purchase as flaxmeal. But beware, they go rancid quickly, so keep ground flax seed (or flaxmeal) in the freezer. Also, it's best to eat in foods that aren't cooked like cereals, sandwiches, salads, and dressings, or with smoothies.

Bountiful beans

Beans are high in protein, fiber, folate, and iron — all beneficial nutrients to promote digestion, lower cholesterol, optimize metabolic rate, and keep you satisfied. You really can't go wrong with the beans you choose to add to your meals. By adding a 1-cup serving to your day, you'll meet about half your fiber and a quarter of your protein needs.

Beans are the best source of *resistant starch*, a type of starch that acts like fiber in your digestive tract. Resistant starch has a great effect on your blood sugar levels; research shows it improves insulin sensitivity. It also acts like a probiotic in a way by promoting healthy bacteria in the gut. Just another reason to make room for beans in your diet!

Beans are known for causing gas, so if that has prevented you from eating them in the past, try this: Wash uncooked beans and soak them overnight in water to soften the skin and release the gas-causing oligosaccharides. You can also boil them and replace the water a couple of times to speed this process up but either way, the beans should be double in size.

If you're not eating them because you don't know how to incorporate them, no more excuses:

✔ Blend chickpeas (garbanzo beans) into hummus and pair with veggies or whole-wheat crackers.

✔ Have edamame (soy beans) as a snack or as an appetizer when you go out to a Japanese restaurant.

✔ Choose lentil soup for a filling snack or meal, and choose white beans to make a classic *pasta e fagioli* soup.

✔ Toss kidney beans into your salad for an extra protein and fiber kick.

✔ Use black beans in any Mexican recipe such as homemade tacos, burritos, or as a side paired with brown rice.

Although canned beans are more convenient than dried, they typically pack sodium, and the lining of the can probably contains the pesticide BPA, which might negatively affect your health. Choose dried beans when time allows for it and cook them in bulk. You can freeze cooked beans so that they stay fresh for months.

Nourishing Nutrients and Supplements

Although I'm a big fan of choosing "food first" when it comes to metabolism-boosting nutrients, because absorption is typically best in food form, I know it's tough to always eat like a nutrition all-star. In this section, I review the main vitamins and minerals that are beneficial for your metabolism. I talk about how to get them in food, if you're able to, how much you need, and when to take a supplement instead.

Always speak with your doctor before taking a vitamin or mineral supplement because it could interact with medication you're taking, be bad for your health in large quantities over a long period of time, or just be plain unnecessary. Also, your body can't use excess nutrients, so many of them will pass through your body unabsorbed, creating, as I've heard it called, "expensive urine."

The main three: Multivitamin, calcium plus D, and fish oil

When it comes to taking supplements, a multivitamin, calcium, vitamin D3, and fish oil are really the only ones I ever recommend (see Table 5-4). It's easy to be drawn into marketing ploys that certain vitamins will give you more energy or that they're formulated to improve your metabolism. Remember, getting the nutrients from foods is best for your energy. There's no such thing as a magic pill for weight loss or metabolism boosting. But in general, you might not be getting all the nutrients you need, and taking a supplement can help prevent deficiencies and protect your health.

Table 5-4   Taking a Multivitamin, Calcium + D, and Fish Oil

The Supplement	The Why	The How
Multivitamin	If your diet isn't varied or you aren't eating enough in general	Once per day with food
Calcium	If you're lactose-intolerant, vegan, or concerned about your bone health	500 milligrams at a time (your body can't absorb more than that). Aim for at least 1,000 milligrams per day between food and supplements.
Vitamin D	If you're taking calcium, vitamin D optimizes its absorption and use by your body.	400-2000 IU per day
Fish oil	If you don't eat fish	Choose a reputable brand with tested purity

With any supplement, defer to your physician to check that it's not interacting with your medication or is counter-productive to your personal health goals.

The rest of the section outlines how other vitamins and minerals affect your metabolic rate. You don't necessarily need to take these as supplements, especially if you are already taking a multivitamin. This info will just give you an idea of how many nutrients are in the metabolism-boosting foods and the many ways they help your burn rate.

B vitamins

The B vitamins include B6, B12, folate, thiamin, and niacin. B vitamins are key players in metabolism and help keep your energy levels high. When your body is deprived of them, you're more likely to feel fatigue and depression, and your metabolism might be sluggish. But megadoses won't boost your rate as the clever marketing on vitamin products would have you believe.

If you're trying to get pregnant or in your child-bearing years, you should be taking folate at the recommended value of 400 micrograms per day to help reduce the risk of neural tube defects in your infant. These occur in the first three weeks after conception, before you know you're pregnant. Therefore, the folate in the prenatal vitamin you start taking once you find out, isn't good enough.

Getting B vitamins from foods, where they work together with other vitamins and minerals, helps optimize their impact. Choose dark, leafy green vegetables like spinach and broccoli, enriched and whole-grain breads, fortified cereals, meat, fish, poultry, and eggs for a variety of those important Bs.

Vitamin D

Vitamin D might be one of the most discussed supplements of the decade because many populations are deficient in it due to decreased sun exposure. Main dietary sources include fatty fish like salmon, mackerel, and canned tuna, eggs, fortified milk, orange juice, cereals, and baby formula. But gaps between what we get and what we need (about 400 international units [IU] per day; 1 IU = 0.025 micrograms of Vitamin D) are remedied by sun exposure, which converts vitamin D into its active form. However, very young children, the elderly, anyone in a northern climate, and those with dark skin are not getting enough sun for their bodies to use the inactive form of vitamin D from foods. Wearing sunscreen also prevents Vitamin D conversion.

Vitamin D is important for calcium absorption and utilization by bones for healthy development, but it's also needed by every tissue in the body, including your precious calorie-burning muscle tissue. In addition, because vitamin D helps make sure your calcium levels are normal, not getting enough can impact your ability to burn fat, leaving more fat ready for storage.

Recently, research also found that vitamin D may help prevent against cancer and heart disease. This isn't an excuse to sit out in the sun all day without sun screen — that puts you at risk for skin cancer. Experts suggest about ten minutes out in the sun midday will do the vitamin D trick. Too much vitamin D can also be toxic, so if you're concerned about your exposure or needs, speak with your doctor.

Magnesium

Most Americans aren't getting enough magnesium. This is a mineral involved in many processes and by every cell in your body. It affects your heart, nerve, and muscle functions, helps keep blood sugar levels stable, and normalizes blood pressure. Magnesium is also a key player in protein synthesis and energy metabolism — that's a lot for one mineral! Although most people aren't getting enough, deficiencies are rarely seen with physical symptoms. But emerging research suggests having enough body stores of magnesium can actually be protective against heart disease and boost immunity.

Magnesium is found in the germ and bran of whole grains, which is removed with refined products. You need about 350 milligrams a day, but getting a variety of whole grains, nuts, fruits, and veggies will ensure you're getting enough. Stock up on these high-in-magnesium foods: wheat bran, almonds, spinach, soybeans, nuts, peanut butter, and oatmeal.

Iron, copper, and zinc

Are you familiar with this trio of metals and essential nutrients that you need to get in your diet?

Iron

You're probably most familiar with iron. Iron carries oxygen through your body by hemoglobin, which is important for every cell. If you don't have enough iron — because you've gone vegan, for example, and aren't getting meat or other products containing iron — and have iron deficiency anemia, your cells won't be getting the oxygen they need, your metabolism will be more sluggish, and your energy will be low. When your energy is low, you'll be less likely to want to exercise or be active, so it's a double whammy. Your burn rate will be even lower.

Men need about 8 milligrams of iron per day, and woman need 18 milligrams per day (to compensate for losses during menstruation) until menopause — after menopause, your needs drop back down to 8 milligrams a day. There are both heme and non-heme sources of iron. *Heme* irons are from animals and are better absorbed in the body. *Non-heme* irons are mainly from plant sources, and absorption can be increased with the addition of vitamin C.

These are the most metabolism-friendly sources of iron and how to make sure it's absorbed:

- ✔ **Heme:** Oysters, turkey, lean ground beef, sirloin, light tuna canned in water, chicken
- ✔ **Non-heme:** Fortified cereal and oatmeals, tofu, spinach, and beans like soybeans, lentils, kidney, lima, blackeyed peas, navy, black, pinto
- ✔ **Enhances iron absorption:** Animal protein and vitamin C (drink orange juice or eat an orange with iron sources or supplements)
- ✔ **Inhibits iron absorption:** Tannins (found in teas) and calcium (don't drink tea or milk, to maximize iron absorption)

Copper

Copper helps the body make the hemoglobin that carries oxygen through your body. Copper also boosts absorption of iron and is an important component of enzymes that have roles in energy production. Copper is found in nutritious foods like seafood, nuts and nut butters, seeds, and beans. You need 900 micrograms daily, 1,000 micrograms during pregnancy, and 1,300 micrograms when breastfeeding.

Zinc

Zinc is an important player in immunity and nerve function and may help lower blood sugar and insulin levels. It also stimulates the pituitary to produce thyroid-stimulating hormone (TSH), so if you're struggling to lose weight because of hypothyroid, zinc could help. It also plays a role in stimulating leptin, so being deficient in zinc can result in a greater appetite. Best food sources include shellfish like oysters, beef, pork, chicken, and baked beans. If you're a vegetarian or vegan, you want to consider a zinc supplement or make sure it's present in your daily multivitamin. Taking zinc supplements can have serious side effects, so do so under the care of your physician. Men need 11 milligrams a day, women 8 milligrams, pregnant women 11 milligrams, and if you're lactating, 12 milligrams.

Spice It Up!

Who said eating healthy has to be boring or bland? Adding herbs and spices to your meals can not only add a pleasure factor to a dish, they may also help increase your metabolic rate. That's not to say these are miracle seeds to sprinkle on your dish and negate the need to make nutritious choices. But if you're choosing foods that are jam-packed with nutrition, staying within your calorie needs, and incorporating these flavors, research has shown herbs and spices can help up your burn rate and improve your health.

Chili pepper and capsaicin

Do you tend to shy away from spicy foods? Maybe this will change your tune — capsaicin, the component of chili peppers that causes the burning sensation in your mouth, also stokes your metabolic fire. A study published in *Obesity* found that capsaicin increases thermogenesis, which releases heat and increases your body temperature, which is why you might break a sweat with a spicy meal. That means it's increasing your metabolic rate — by up to 50 percent for 3 hours after the meal, according to one study. Research out of Thailand also found that capsaicin has the potential to lower blood sugar levels.

Try experimenting and incorporating more heat into your meals. It's an acquired taste; you'll be able to tolerate more and more heat, and then might need more of it to achieve the same metabolic shift.

Common chili peppers include bell peppers, cayenne peppers, pepperoncini, jalapenos, and habaneros (warning: not for beginners):

✔ Slice peppers over salads; add to soups, stews, or side dishes.

✔ Grind them into dips, such as guacamole and salsas, spreads, and salad dressings.

✔ Dried chilis are ground into powders, which you can add as a dry rub for meats, fish, tofu, and vegetables.

✔ Use chipotle hot sauce over anything like eggs, in sandwiches, on rice dishes, with desserts — basically anything you like!

Ginger

Ginger is a spice found in many forms — pickled with your sushi, in some brands of ginger ale, in the form of candy, dried for addition to dishes, and added to tea and smoothies. It's been used for centuries in many cultures to help calm digestion and for numerous other ailments. Recently, animal studies have found that ginger can increase metabolism by up to 20 percent, but its main benefit to you is its antioxidant content and ability to increase gastric juices to promote good digestion. Ginger has also been extensively studied for reducing nausea during pregnancy morning sickness and during chemotherapy.

Turmeric

Turmeric is the plant material that you might recognize in curries when it's ground into a deep orange-yellow powder. Curcumin, the active component of turmeric, has been shown to have anti-inflammatory and anti-cancer benefits. Animal studies have also noted a reduction in fat storage with curcumin, but as with many spices and herbs, more research is needed to really understand the effects. That said, it certainly can't hurt to include turmeric into your repertoire if you like the flavor. Look for curry powders and check for turmeric in the ingredient to add as flavoring to main dishes like tofu, chicken, fish, and sides like vegetables.

Cinnamon

Cinnamon has been in the spotlight lately for people with diabetes. It's been shown to help diabetics reduce their hemoglobin A1C level — a reflection of blood glucose levels over the past few months — as well as reduce cholesterol and blood pressure. It's possible that cinnamon works by helping insulin work more effectively. The most consistent effect cinnamon has had across the board is improving fasting blood glucose levels and, subsequently, spikes in your hunger levels. Its benefits are controversial. By no means should cinnamon replace any other diabetes treatment, but there are certainly some promising studies. Cinnamon is also delicious: Add it to oatmeal, skim lattes, and apple slices. You can also add it to curries for a double dose of power spices.

Green tea

Although not exactly a spice, green tea is worth mentioning for its researched ability to increase fat oxidation and boost thermogenesis up to 4 percent. The studies are limited. But because green tea contains antioxidants (called *polyphenols*) and flavonoids (called *catechins*), which fight disease and decrease inflammation, it's definitely a crowd pleaser when it comes to health. Drink green tea hot or iced, but remember, it does contain caffeine, although only about ½ as much as black tea and ¼ as much as coffee, you still want to limit your intake close to bedtime.

Should You Buy Organic?

According to *Consumer Reports*, at least two thirds of Americans consumed an organic food within the past year, and spending on organic foods has increased about 20 percent each year over the past decade. In 2011, the organic food sector generated close to 30 billion dollars. At the same time, consumers continue to be confused about what *organic* means and get it mixed up with definitions for foods that are *local* and *natural*. That's a lot of funds generated in the name of organic foods, when consumers can't tell you what *organic* even means. Because you can expect to shell out 50–100 percent more money for organic products versus conventional counterparts, you'll want to know if it's really worth it.

What does organic mean anyway?

According to the National Organic Program of the USDA (2012), the definition of organic is as follows:

> *"Organic is a labeling term that indicates that the food or other agricultural product has been produced through approved methods. These methods integrate cultural, biological, and mechanical practices that foster cycling of resources, promote ecological balance, and conserve biodiversity. Synthetic fertilizers, sewage sludge, irradiation, and genetic engineering may not be used."*

In the most basic terms, then, organic foods are not grown using synthetic fertilizers and pesticides. The animals can't be given any hormones to promote growth or antibiotics to prevent disease. The cost of adhering to these methods, including more manpower, and the fact that the yield is iffier, gets transferred to the consumer.

Foods that adhere to these standards receive organic certification and may use the label shown in Figure 5-1.Unless the food package reads "100% organic," the organic label indicates the product contains 95 percent organic ingredients. There's also a "Made with organic ingredients" designation that uses even fewer organic ingredients, 70–94 percent.

Figure 5-1: USDA Organic label. Food must contain 95 percent organic ingredients.

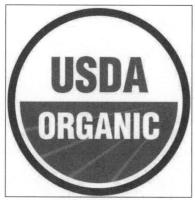

Image courtesy of USDA. See www.ams.usda.gov.

What does this mean for your health? A recent review of studies over the past 50 years conducted in London found that organic foods were not necessarily nutritionally superior.

How bad are pesticides?

Pesticides are used in farming to prevent crop destruction by bacteria, insects, or other animals. But just because a food is organic doesn't mean there are no pesticides in it. It means that the pesticides used are derived from natural sources, not synthetic material. When it comes to synthetic pesticides, the jury is out on how they really affect people. It's possible that these chemicals may contribute to obesity, cancer, and other diseases. But I don't want to be an alarmist about it, because there's not enough substantial research about how risky exposure to these chemicals really is. The studies exposing an increased risk of obesity have been conducted in rats with exposure thousands of times higher than what people eat. One study in *Environmental Health Perspectives* found that exposure to pesticides in children may impact brain development. But the FDA monitors levels of the pesticides in our food and deems certain types safe for human consumption. And there's not much research on the health of people who primarily consume organic foods. I bring it up because these chemicals aren't natural. Your body might not be so adept at processing them, which could potentially affect your metabolic rate and your health.

As far as the nutrient content of produce, the main determinant is really travel and handling time between when the plant is picked and when you eat it. Nutrients are lost during that time, and just because a food is organic, it doesn't mean it's locally produced. It can travel the same distance as conventional products. Also, organic products can be high in sodium and saturated fat, so you still need to be an educated consumer and read the Nutrition Facts label.

When to go organic

Whether or not you decide to choose organic foods is a personal choice. You have to weigh the possible benefits and costs of the added expense. If you can afford to support farmers who choose these more environmentally friendly methods, that's definitely a solid reason to go organic as well.

The Environmental Working Group (EWG) has come up with The Dirty Dozen: 12 types of produce that have the highest level of pesticides. So, use your "organic dollars" on these foods first instead of buying all organic foods. Also because children's bodies are growing at a rapid rate, you might want to limit young children's exposure to these conventional products.

The reasons the following are higher in pesticides are due to more permeable skins with bigger pores for the chemical to get in, or the methods in which they are grown:

- ✔ Peaches
- ✔ Apples
- ✔ Sweet Bell peppers
- ✔ Celery
- ✔ Nectarines
- ✔ Strawberries
- ✔ Cherries
- ✔ Pears
- ✔ Grapes (imported)
- ✔ Spinach
- ✔ Lettuce
- ✔ Potatoes

Not only produce is affected by pesticides. Animal products such as meat, dairy, fish, and eggs contain pesticides too, along with hormones, antibiotics, and insecticides.

Deciphering label terms

Along with organic seals of approval, you'll see these other voluntary terms on foods labels for livestock products like meat and eggs. Regarding the ethical and fair treatment of animals, here's what these USDA-regulated terms mean:

- ✔ **Free Range:** Flock was provided shelter but had continuous access to the outdoors and unlimited access to food and fresh water. This is regulated by the USDA.

- ✔ **Cage Free:** Flock could roam freely in a building, room, or enclosure, with unlimited access to food and fresh water during their production cycle.

- ✔ **Natural:** Meat, poultry, and egg products bearing a *natural* label must be minimally processed without artificial ingredients. This doesn't pertain to products that don't contain meat and eggs, nor does it have anything to do with farming practices.

- ✔ **Grass Fed:** These animals receive majority of nutrients from grass throughout their lives, which tends to result in higher levels of omega-3 fatty acids, antioxidants, and conjugated linoleic acid (CLA), which have been studied for benefits in weight management and protection against cancer. Remember this label doesn't limit use of antibiotics, hormones, or pesticides, unless labeled "grass-fed organic."

To minimize your pesticide exposure, look for organic labels on these products. One note on that: Only farm-raised fish can technically qualify as organic, because their food intake is controlled. However, farm-raised fish are typically higher in other contaminants such as mercury and heavy metals. So I'd suggest skipping organic fish and going for wild whenever possible.

When not to bother going organic

Many fruits and vegetables don't absorb too many chemicals as they grow, and some aren't sprayed as much with pesticides if they don't attract insects. The EWG has also come up with 12 cleanest pieces of produce you can choose conventionally, to save pressure on your wallet from purchasing organic:

- ✔ Onions
- ✔ Avocado
- ✔ Sweet corn
- ✔ Pineapples
- ✔ Mango
- ✔ Asparagus
- ✔ Sweet peas
- ✔ Kiwi
- ✔ Bananas
- ✔ Cabbage
- ✔ Broccoli
- ✔ Papaya

No product will be completely devoid of chemical residue, so always wash your fruits and vegetables with water — even fruit with inedible skins, because once you cut the surface, pesticides can be transferred from you knife to the pulp inside. Also, pesticides accumulate in fat, so with meats, trim fat and remove the skin to reduce not just saturated fat but your intake of pesticides.

Chapter 6

Planning Meals: Composition, Timing, and Eating Behavior

In This Chapter

▶ Understanding how to eat to boost your rate

▶ Identifying true hunger and what to do when it's not true hunger

▶ Learning how to plan your meals with sample ideas

*Y*our food habits — the way you eat and think about eating — didn't develop overnight. They were created and started evolving as early as your first or second year of life. It's easy to get frustrated when you're trying to make healthy changes, and it takes a while to get them to stick. But you have to first be realistic (if you're not sure how, flip back to Chapter 4) and then be patient with yourself when breaking old habits.

This chapter focuses on making behavioral changes to boost your metabolic rate. Although the composition of your diet counts, the *how* is often more challenging because of the way you've been eating for years. The changes you need to focus on include the following:

✔ Timing of your meals

✔ Portion sizes

✔ Your ability to obey your physical hunger cues

Also, certain combinations of foods actually can help your metabolic rate so that you feel satisfied and reap the most nutrition you can from those foods.

Planning ahead sets you up for success when it comes to making decisions. You're more likely to choose something healthy if you've thought it out ahead of time or stocked that choice for easy access. Common sense? Maybe so. But many find planning ahead to be a huge time commitment and use that as an excuse to stick to old habits. I promise, it doesn't have to be so hard (then again, if it were super easy, everyone would do it). In this chapter, I give you examples of how you can plan ahead. I also offer up sample meal plans to get you started on your way to a healthier metabolism.

Eating Less, More Frequently

I don't really like the concept of food rules, and I'm not trying to be the diet police, but eating a meal or snack every 3 to 4 hours is something that is integral to keeping your metabolism moving all day long. If you're someone who has one big meal at the end of the day, be aware that spreading those calories out more throughout the day can help your metabolism, improve your energy, and reduce your stress levels.

When you go many hours between meals, here's what happens:

- ✔ Your metabolism can slow down because it's not being fueled regularly. Then it wises up to this, and after a few days, to compensate, might not burn calories off as effectively.

- ✔ You're more likely to be ravenous, lowering your inhibitions to make unhealthy choices at the next meal.

- ✔ Your blood sugar levels drop, you're cranky, and you have food cravings (like when you hit up your office vending machine at 4 p.m.).

- ✔ You can feel more anxious and tired without a steady supply of nutrients to fuel your body and mind. You also have less energy to exercise harder or longer, which, in turn, affects your metabolic rate.

 If you have difficulty remembering to eat, try setting an alert on your phone as a reminder. If you want to get even more specific, you can even include in the reminder what you're going to eat at that time. Some smartphone apps such as FoodRemindr, Eat 'N Sleep, and Simple Meal Reminder, will let you set up notifications as well with less effort.

The amount that you eat at each of these meals and snacks is up to you, as long as it's within your calorie allotment for the day. I consider a snack to be about 100–300 calories and a meal 300–700 calories or more, but honestly, it's really up to you to decide what's going to be practical with your lifestyle and how hungry you feel.

Some people graze all day, eat about 200 calories every 2–3 hours and that works for them as far as energy supply and staying within calorie needs. But that can be impractical if you can't think about food frequently when you're at work or on-the-go. Also grazing can have downfalls: Each time you eat you may not feel as satisfied as you do when you eat a meal or more substantial snack, which results in overeating later on or not having the energy you need to get through your day. It'll be trial and error for you to see what works best for you personally. There's no proven benefit to either strategy, and in the sample meal plans later on in this chapter, you'll see how you can mix it up with different calorie intakes and timing of meals depending on what's practical for you.

Is late-night eating bad for you?

Have you done the no-eating-after-8 p.m. diet? Many people are under the impression that if you eat something late at night, it'll be more likely to go to your hips than if you ate it midday. The truth is that your body is constantly digesting and burning calories, even overnight, so any time of day you eat it, it will be broken down and stored the same way.

In my experience, clients who stop eating at night can be successful, but typically it's because they were not eating much during the day and were then overeating late at night or emotional-eating when stressed or bored at home. A study published in *Obesity* found that night owls consume about 248 more calories each day than those who have an earlier bedtime, and most of those are consumed in the evening. Also, the types of foods people typically consume at night are snacky high-fat foods. These types of foods can interfere with having the best sleep possible, which, in turn, throws off your hormone balance. Research shows that each of our organs contains circadian clocks which possibly dictate times of day when digestion is best, during waking periods. But if you're getting your 7–8 hours of sleep, eating the right foods, and spreading your calories throughout the day, there's no need to hyper-focus on not eating after a certain time at night.

Having a snack at night is important if you eat dinner early and are up late, especially if you have diabetes and you need to maximize blood sugar control. As long as you're choosing the right types of snacks and moderate your portions, you'll be good to go. Good options at night include:

- ¾ cup whole grain cereal with ½ cup low-fat milk
- ½ apple sliced with 1–2 tablespoons peanut butter
- 4 ounces low-fat yogurt with 1 cup melon
- ½ whole grain pita with ¼ cup low-fat shredded cheese, 2 tablespoons tomato sauce — heated up!

Combinations of foods are the most important piece of this equation (more on this later in the chapter). If you're just eating gummy bears all day, which are straight simple sugar, you'll be having spikes in your blood glucose, dips in your energy, and you'll never feel satisfied. If you like gummy bears and want to have a serving, you need to pair it with what I like to call a *curber*, a food that contains fiber, lean protein, or heart-healthy fats. This more nutritious food will help curb the impact of the sugar spike and your hunger.

Eat Breakfast, No Excuses!

The first meal of the day is called *breakfast* because you're literally breaking a fast of many hours without food. Your metabolism is moving less overnight when you're sleeping because you're not physically active or eating. When you wake up, you want to eat something within a few hours so that you wake up your metabolism too. That gets you geared up to digest and use food for fuel all day long.

If you skip breakfast, you're more likely to replace those calories with more snacking or bigger meals throughout the day, be overweight, and meet less of your *micronutrient* needs (nutrients like vitamins and minerals that are required in small amounts by the body for metabolism and growth) throughout the day. Not only do breakfast eaters start the day off on a healthy note with a balanced meal, they're also more likely to do the following:

- ✔ **Lose weight and keep it off:** People who eat breakfast eat less throughout the day and have 30 percent lower overweight/obesity rates. Also, 78 percent of people in the National Weight Control Registry report eating breakfast every day. These are people who have lost at least 30 pounds and successfully maintained their weight for a minimum of one year. 90 percent eat breakfast at least 5 days per week.

- ✔ **Meet nutrient needs:** People who skip breakfast are less likely to get their daily requirements of fiber and calcium. Because breakfast is a good opportunity to get whole-grain cereals, fruits, milk, and yogurt, people who skip might consume less of these foods. And people make more nutritious choices all day long with a balanced breakfast.

- ✔ **Exercise:** Breakfast eaters are more likely to make time for exercise during the day. Maybe you have more energy to be active or you're up early exercising and, therefore, eat breakfast. Whichever it is, these two behaviors are linked.

- ✔ **Be more focused:** Studies find that children have better attention spans and memory skills in school with a solid breakfast in them. This is true for adults, too. I know that I'm personally a waste of time and not as productive in the morning without breakfast.

If you never eat breakfast, start small. If it's because you don't feel hunger, maybe you're eating too much late at night. Break the cycle of not eating much during the day and nighttime overeating. Start small and build up to something more substantial as you get into a routine. Having a combination of lean protein and fiber is particularly important in the morning to keep you satisfied until lunchtime. These nutrients take long to digest, help prevent blood glucose spikes, and fill you up most effectively.

Here are some ideas:

- ✔ If you typically have corn flakes, switch to a high-fiber cereal and/or add berries to your bowl.

- ✔ If you already eat oatmeal, top with a serving of chopped nuts or pair with a hard-cooked egg for a dose of protein.

✔ If you have a muffin, eat half (it's probably too big) and add a "curber" like low-fat yogurt to round it out.

✔ If you normally have a bagel, switch to two slices of whole wheat bread with peanut butter and sliced banana (my personal favorite).

✔ If you only have coffee, build up with, first, a piece of fruit, then a serving of yogurt, and then mix in high-fiber cereal for a healthy parfait.

✔ If you need something to bring with you on-the-go, whip up a smoothie with fruit, low-fat dairy, or soy milk. (Find recipes for this and other nutritious breakfast options in Chapter 7.)

Power Combinations of Foods

Although the metabolism-boosting foods of Chapter 5 are nutritious on their own, pairing foods together can maximize their potential. Having a balance among your meals helps you get all the nutrients you need and keeps your metabolic rate high.

The previous section mentions how pairing fiber and protein at breakfast is great for satiation, and that's also true for lunch, snack, and dinner. If you fully round out that meal with an unsaturated fat, you'll enhance that effect even further. Not only that, but making healthy choices within the *macronutrient* (types of food required in large amounts by the body like protein, fat, and carbohydrate) groups can help boost your immunity and reduce your risk for diseases.

Most frequently, I see meals containing foods that have a high percentage of carbohydrate without much protein or fat to balance out the plate. For example, a plate of pasta with vegetables — although the meal has nutritious components, it's missing protein and fat to fuel your digestion. Adding grilled chicken or beans can help fill you up and consume a smaller portion overall.

In addition to balancing your plate, try these power pairs of foods for a healthy bonus:

✔ **Add avocado to your salad.** Research shows that heart-healthy fats paired with tomatoes and dark leafy green vegetables can help absorption of the antioxidants within, such as lycopene (protective against cancer) and lutein (protects your eyes). Also, just eating tomatoes and spinach or broccoli together helps boost lycopene's power.

✔ **Make a fruit salad with berries and apples.** The quercetin found in berries and the catechins in apples (actually apples contain both) work together to improve platelet clotting and may prevent cardiac events like heart attacks.

✔ **Cook up a side of beans laced with greens.** Non-heme iron found in beans is better absorbed when paired with a dose of vitamin C, such as with kale, spinach, or broccoli.

✔ **Steel-cut oatmeal and orange juice.** Phenols, antioxidant compounds, in the oatmeal and vitamin C in the OJ, work together to reduce your LDL or "bad" cholesterol to improve heart health.

✔ **Spice up your salmon.** Turmeric, the spice that gives curry powder it's bright orange-yellow coloring, and the omega-3 in fish may doubly protect against cancer by preventing cells from multiplying. Although fatty fish on its own has the potential to improve heart health, adding turmeric can boost this effect.

✔ **Blend a smoothie with nuts or seeds and skim milk**. While you may choose skim milk to reduce your saturated fat intake, you do need fat for absorption of vitamins like vitamin D and vitamin A found in the milk. In your smoothie, add a serving of walnuts or flaxseeds for a boost and a more satisfying drink.

Overcoming Portion Distortion

Many people believe that oversized portions are the reason a third of Americans are overweight or obese, but the reasons for the epidemic are multifaceted and that's a discussion which could fill up a whole other book. But it's true that as American's waistlines have expanded since the 1970s, portion sizes and the size of our plates have grown consistently as well (not to mention rates of diabetes and heart disease). According to the Centers for Disease Control (CDC), over the past 50 years

✔ Fast-food burgers have tripled in size, from 4 ounces (300 calories) to 12 ounces (850 calories).

✔ The average order of fries went from 2.4 ounces (217 calories) to 6.7 ounces (600 calories).

✔ Soft drinks are rarely offered at 7 ounces (85 calories) and are now frequently ordered at 42 ounces (509 calories).

Those are significant increases! Even if you only made one mega-portion order every time you went out to eat, that would correlate to 6 pounds added per year, assuming you only go out to eat *once* per week. Not only have fast-food sizes increased, all types of foods are larger. Bagels have doubled in size from 3 to 6 inches in diameter, adding about 200 calories to your morning meal. Recipes that used to make 24 servings in cookbooks decades ago now only allow you to make a fraction of that amount simply due to the fact that consumers are used to larger portions.

Mindless eating affects portions

When supersized portions look normal to you, you're much more likely to eat more and think less about what you're eating. Brian Wansink, a professor from my alma mater Cornell University and author of *Mindless Eating* (Bantam, 2010), has conducted fascinating research on the topic.

One study involved stale (5-day old!) popcorn, which he provided to moviegoers in either medium or supersize large containers. People who had the larger buckets ate, on average 53 percent more than those with the medium buckets throughout the course of the movie, even if they had just eaten lunch beforehand. The bottom line is that the moviegoers didn't eat because they were hungry, or because the popcorn tasted particularly good. They ate because it was there, and ate more if it was in a bigger container.

In other studies, including one testing a group of nutritionists, Wansink found that people served themselves about 30 percent more when given a larger bowl or plate to dish out on. The exact reason for these correlations isn't clear, but by being aware of your environment and manipulating how you eat, you'll be better able to control your portions.

One way to manipulate your eating environment is to make it more stress-free and enjoyable by dimming the lights, lighting candles, and playing soothing music. In one of his recent studies, published in *Psychology Reports* in September 2012, Wansink found that diners in this mood lighting with soft music ate about 18 percent less than those in the uncontrolled environment. He found that these diners were more happy and satisfied with their meals.

One reason portion sizes have grown is that if you're offered bang for your buck, you'll buy the larger size. For example, if an Italian restaurant gives you double the typical serving of pasta, but only charges you $2 more, you're happy with the value. You could come out the victor if you took half home in a doggy bag for another meal, but the issue is that you probably don't and end up eating more instead.

Research shows that people underestimate what they eat by up to 200 percent when out to eat and that a dinner plate is 23 percent larger (from 9.6 inches to 11.8 inches in diameter) than it was 50 years ago. Portions sizes are not only blown out of proportion in restaurants, but also in packaged foods for sale in the grocery store and in vending machines everywhere.

The definitions of *portion size* and *serving size* are two different measurements. A serving size as listed on a food label as equal to a standardized unit of food, not necessarily what's in the entire package if you ate it all (the portion). For example, if a bag of trail mix says it provides three "servings," you should take the number of calories the label says are in a "serving" and multiply that by three. If you typically eat half the bag, multiply that total number by two for the amount of calories in your "portion." It's okay to have more than one serving per meal as long as you're staying within a total amount for the day. When you're out to eat, use Table 6-1 to eyeball what a serving size is just to esti-mate. For even more tips on how to stick to healthy habits when dining out, check out Chapter 14.

Table 6-1	Common Measurements for Food Servings	
Food	*Serving*	*Measure*
Fruit/vegetable	½ cup fresh	Tennis ball
Poultry, meat, fish	3 ounces	Deck of cards
Grains	½ cup cooked	Size of your fist
Baked potato	3 ounces	Small computer mouse
Cheese	1 ounce	4 dice stacked
Nuts, nut butter, hummus	1 ounce	Ping pong ball
Pancake/waffle	1 ounce	Compact disc
Bagel	1 ounce	Hockey puck
Oil	1 teaspoon	Poker chip

When at home, controlling the environment is key to managing your portion sizes:

✓ When you purchase foods in bulk, portion out servings into smaller containers for easy grab-and-go eating.

✓ Never eat out of the big bag of chips (or other food). Pre-portion a serving into a small bowl and put the bigger container away.

✓ Stock your refrigerator with nutritious foods like single pieces of fruits and cut-up vegetables to nosh on.

✓ Use a scale to measure the weight to gauge how much you're eating for foods without labels.

✓ Use smaller plates — 10 inches — but not less than that because you might be tempted to go for seconds.

✓ Make your eating environment less stressful by putting aside at least 30 minutes to eat a meal. Create a place setting and replace loud television noise with soft music so you'll eat more slowly and be more satisfied.

Are You Really Hungry?

The most important question to ask yourself before eating is whether you really have physical hunger — call it stomach hunger. When you were younger, you probably listened to your body and ate when you were hungry and stopped when you were full. But throughout the years, you may have started using food as a way to fill another type of void emotionally or correlated foods to certain memories, occasions, and people that make you more likely to overeat. When you want to eat for other reasons besides needing nutrients, call it *mouth hunger*.

Distinguishing between the two types of hunger isn't so easy after you've ignored your physical hunger cues all of these years. Signs of stomach hunger, or that you have gone too long without food, include the following:

✔ Stomach gurgling or discomfort

✔ Irritability

✔ Shaking

✔ Light-headedness or headache

Signs of mouth or emotional hunger include the following:

✔ Urge to eat in response to anxiety, stress, sadness, loneliness, boredom

✔ Being insatiable no matter what you've eaten

✔ Responding to a desire to control weight or improve appearance

✔ Eating more than normal during a happy occasion or holiday

Being more in tune with your physical hunger can help you get back to the mentality you had as a child, using food for fuel and not as a solution for emotions. We all know that food won't solve our problems and, in fact, will spur feelings of shame after hitting up the refrigerator late at night. And so it becomes a vicious cycle.

Here are two ideas about how to start recognizing your stomach hunger and breaking out of that emotional eating cycle:

✔ **Rate your hunger**: Use a scale from 0–10, where 0 means absolutely starving and 10 is uncomfortably full. Eat when you're at a 2 or 3, stop at a 7 or 8.

✔ **Take the apple test**: If you think you're *mouth hungry* and crave something salty or sweet, ask yourself, could I eat an apple right now? If so, eat the apple (or any fruit) or nosh on cut-up veggies to reap those nutrients. If the answer is no, you may just be "emotionally hungry" and need to quell that with something besides food. Make a list of the activities you enjoy doing that can substitute for these emotions. Physically writing them down and posting inside your kitchen cabinet can be more powerful than keeping in your head.

The more time you put between the desire to eat and eating, the better. Cravings come in waves, so when you find yourself in the kitchen, and you're unsure how you got there, distract yourself with a healthy activity (ideas coming up), and it's possible the craving will pass. If it doesn't, do another activity. If it still doesn't, you might be physically hungry and need to eat a snack:

- ✔ **If you're sad or lonely:** Call a friend or a family member, go to a group exercise class in the evening, or go for walks around your neighborhood. A study out of Duke University found that people following an aerobic exercise regimen required less prescription medication for depression. If you need additional support, seek out help from a mental health professional (more on that in Chapter 13).

- ✔ **If you're stressed or anxious**: Soothe yourself with a bath, practice deep breathing or stretching movements, listen to your favorite music, reorganize your closet, or keep a journal. If you're angry, keeping a journal can be particularly helpful to letting out that emotion. You can also try writing a letter to the person or thing you're angry or stressed about (but don't send it)!

- ✔ **If you're bored**: Keep your hands busy by reading a book, knitting or engaging in another hobby, fixing things, cleaning around the house, or (my personal favorite for the ladies) painting your nails — you won't want to mess those up by fumbling through the snacks in your pantry.

Don't just shovel food into your mouth. It takes at least 20 minutes for your brain to get the signal that your stomach is full. You'll experience more satisfaction from a food mentally as well if you slow down and savor it and create an enjoyable environment to eat in.

Sample Meal Plans

In this section, I provide you with meal ideas for a sample week's plan. This is just a guide — I don't expect you to follow what I say exactly. Of course, you can get started on a healthy path, but for any plan to be realistic, it's got to be individualized for you. Therefore, use the information in this section as a jumping-off point to plan your meals ahead. Pick foods that you love and are likely to incorporate without feeling like you're on a restricted *diet*.

You may be surprised to see some of the items in these meal plans. I always emphasize having a balance of foods, both nutritious and fun, so that you don't feel deprived. In general, stick to one fun food per day. By *fun food* I mean one that *isn't* on the metabolism-boosting list but *is* something you love to eat. If you totally avoid the foods you love, your plan won't be sustainable for you in the long term. Remember, this is about a way of life, not a quick fix. If you're satisfied both physically and mentally, you're more likely to be successful.

If one day you happen to have all fun foods, don't beat yourself up. You can get right back to it the next time you have a meal or snack — note, I didn't say tomorrow. The *next time* you're making a food decision, do the next right thing by making it a healthy one. (For more tips on how to cheat the best way you can, check out Chapter 13.)

In these meal plans I don't include complicated recipes. Not everyone cooks, and I believe you don't have to be a master chef to make healthy choices. I also am not including super fancy ingredients that you'll buy once and never use again. These meal plans are focused on practical foods and the basics of balance at each meal/snack, whether you're choosing these foods when out to eat or prepping them in your kitchen. You can also check out the recipes in Part III to get ideas for jazzing up these sample meal plans.

Each day is about 1,500–1,600 calories, but I break the calories down by meal so you can mix and match depending on your needs (to calculate your daily calorie needs, refer to Chapter 3). If you require more calories, add another serving of a whole grain, lean protein, fruit, vegetable, or heart-healthy fat to the meal. Or add another snack to the day. If you require less, take a look at what the lower-in-calorie balanced meals and snacks look like.

The balance among nutrients and not going more than 4 hours between meals are key to stay satisfied and keep your metabolism moving. Therefore, these daily meal plans offer up a variety of solutions, based on when you wake up and go to sleep, and give you options for spreading your calories throughout the day.

Just another manic Monday

- ✔ **Breakfast:** 6 ounces fat-free Greek yogurt, 1 cup blueberries, 1 cup halved strawberries, 2 tablespoons ground flaxseed (300 calories)
- ✔ **Lunch:** Deli-Style Tuna Salad Sandwich (Refer to Chapter 8 for the recipe), 16 baby carrots (350 calories)
- ✔ **Snack:** 1 ounce pistachio nuts (160 calories)
- ✔ **Dinner:** 2 ounces whole-wheat pasta, 3 ounces chicken, 1 cup broccoli, 1 tablespoon olive oil, 4 tablespoons grated parmesan cheese (500 calories)
- ✔ **Dessert:** ½ cup vanilla ice cream (200 calories)

Tasty Tuesday

- ✔ **Breakfast:** 2 scrambled omega-3-fortified eggs, 2 slices whole-grain toast, 1 cup skim milk (400 calories)

- ✔ **Lunch:** Veggie Mexican salad with 2 cups leafy greens, ½ cup sliced tomato, ½ cup black beans, 1 ounce part-skim cheese, 1 ounce avocado, ½ cup sweet corn, 1 tablespoon olive oil (470 calories)

- ✔ **Snack:** 2 large graham crackers with 1 tablespoon nut butter (250 calories)

- ✔ **Dinner:** 4 ounces grilled wild salmon with cayenne pepper rub, small baked sweet potato, 12 spears grilled asparagus (300 calories)

- ✔ **Dessert:** 3 cups air-popped popcorn (100 calories)

Late start Wednesday

- ✔ **Breakfast:** Energizing Citrus Ginger Smoothie (Recipe in Chapter 7) (300 calories)

- ✔ **Lunch:** Chicken and mixed vegetable (red pepper, mushroom, carrots) stir-fry (1 ½ cups) with 1 cup brown rice, side greens salad with 1 tablespoon vinaigrette (500 calories)

- ✔ **Snack:** Orange, 1 ounce dark chocolate (180 calories)

- ✔ **Dinner:** Sirloin Steak Tacos (Get the recipe in Chapter 9) (620 calories)

Trying Vegan Thursday

- ✔ **Breakfast:** Whole-wheat English muffin, 2 tablespoons peanut butter, ½ banana sliced, 1 cup soy milk (450 calories)

- ✔ **Lunch:** Make your own salad: 2 cups romaine lettuce, 5 ounces pomegranate seeds, 1 cup diced firm tofu, ¼ cup chickpeas, 1 radish chopped, ½ cup sliced fennel, 2 tablespoons Italian vinaigrette. 1 cup melon (500 calories)

- ✔ **Snack:** Fruit and nut bar (200 calories)

- ✔ **Dinner:** Veggie burger on whole-grain bun, 1 cup cooked spaghetti squash strands, ½ cup roasted pumpkin seeds (420 calories)

Stay Fit Friday

- ✔ **Breakfast:** 1 cup steel-cut oats, ¼ cup chopped nuts (375 calories)

- ✔ **Lunch:** Waldorf wrap: Multigrain wrap with 3 ounces diced cooked chicken, lettuce, ½ cup diced apples, 7 walnut halves, 1 tablespoon mustard, balsamic vinegar (450 calories)

- ✔ **Snack:** 2 medium oatmeal raisin cookies, 1 glass skim milk (250 calories)

- ✔ **Dinner:** 3 ounce grilled shrimp mixed with ½ cup cooked whole grain (like quinoa), 1 tablespoon olive oil, 1 cup Brussels sprouts (375 calories)

- ✔ **Dessert:** 1 cup banana "ice cream" (only ingredient is blended frozen banana) (150 calories)

A more snacky Saturday

- ✔ **Breakfast:** ¾ cup whole-wheat cereal, 1 cup low-fat milk, 1 cup sectioned grapefruit (3-inch diameter) (300 calories)

- ✔ **Snack:** 1 ½ cup lentil soup with ½ cup spinach (235 calories)

- ✔ **Snack:** ½ turkey sandwich: 3 ounces roast turkey, 1 slice whole-wheat bread. 1 peach (250 calories)

- ✔ **Snack:** Frozen Yogurt Covered Blueberry Bites (Get the recipe in Chapter 10) (120 calories)

- ✔ **Dinner:** 2 slices pizza with whole-wheat crust (each ⅛ of a 14 inch pie), 1 cup braised kale (600 calories)

Sleep-in Sunday

- ✔ **Late breakfast:** 2 whole-wheat pancakes (6-inch diameter), 1 medium fresh peach, sliced, ½ cup low-fat cottage cheese (450 calories)

- ✔ **Lunch:** Spinach salad (2 cups) with 1 hard-cooked egg, ¼ cup dried cranberries, 1 tablespoons pine nuts, vinegar and olive oil (1 tablespoon) and 6 ounces low-fat Greek yogurt mixed with 1 tablespoon dark chocolate chips and cinnamon (500 calories)

- ✔ **Snack:** 4 tablespoons hummus, 1 cup sliced jicama or any crunchy vegetable (150 calories)

- ✔ **Dinner:** Japanese take-out: 1 cup edamame, 1 cup tofu miso soup, 2 rolls tuna and cucumber sushi with brown rice (500 calories)

Early to bed for the week ahead!

 Another piece of the puzzle is stocking your kitchen with metabolism- boosting foods. For more details on this, see my free article "Setting Up Your Kitchen For Success" at http://www.dummies.com/extras/boostingyour metabolism/.

Part III
Recipes

The recipes in this part are designed to be realistic to easily incorporate into your metabolism-boosting lifestyle. No fancy ingredients or complicated methods, just balanced and delicious meals that won't break the calorie bank. But there's more involved in cooking than just throwing together ingredients from a recipe. Check out my bonus online article on setting up a metabolism-boosting kitchen at `www.dummies.com/extras/boostingyourmetabolism/`.

In this part . . .

✔ Start your day the right way with metabolism-boosting breakfasts.

✔ Keep your metabolic rate boosted throughout your day with powerful lunches.

✔ Prepare delicious appetizers, side dishes, and dinners to finish up your day.

✔ Get great ideas on terrific snacks to keep around.

Chapter 7

Awaken Your Metabolism with a Balanced Breakfast

*B*reaking your overnight fast with breakfast is the first line of defense for the day against a sluggish metabolism. No matter what you eat, having breakfast within a few hours of waking up helps wake up your metabolic rate. But like a domino effect, making more nutritious choices and having a balanced breakfast helps you also make healthier choices all day long.

You may rush out the door on the weekdays and grab a donut or bagel to go. Although that's better than nothing, start to incorporate foods rich in fiber like whole grains and fruit, and protein from eggs or low-fat dairy, even heart-healthy fats from nuts and seeds, which provide the best fuel to power you through the day, keep you satisfied, and keep your metabolic rate high.

Having a balance among all those nutrients helps provide you with the most energy to awaken your metabolism for the day. No wonder people who eat breakfast are more likely to lose and maintain their weight loss. Breakfast eaters are also more productive throughout the day, including with exercise, another major part of the metabolism equation.

Wholesome Whole Grains

Breakfast is a great excuse to make room for a serving or two of whole grains because it's the meal most people eat at home. When you're out to dine, it's not guaranteed you'll get your serving of whole grains. The refined grains you get from foods like white bread, pasta, and rice won't offer filling fiber, energizing B vitamins and magnesium, and other nutrients like zinc which help keep your blood sugar more stable. Therefore, choosing whole grains first thing in the morning can help keep you focused and less likely to succumb to cravings all day long.

Quick and Easy Eggs

Eggs are often overlooked as an excellent source of protein, which is heart healthy and wallet friendly. Having protein first thing in the morning helps keep you satisfied until lunchtime. Although having egg yolks, about four per week, is perfectly acceptable (most of the fat within is from unsaturated fat), you don't want to go overboard with the yolks since they do contain cholesterol.

Although it's mainly saturated fat that raises cholesterol in your blood, the cholesterol in food does play a role. So you'll see egg whites used in many of these recipes for beneficial lean protein, without the cholesterol or added fat, and also to cut the calorie count. If you want to use liquid egg whites, use 2 tablespoons per egg white.

Breakfast To-Go

Because you may not have time to cook breakfast every morning, you'll find smoothies, an energy bar, and a Chia Muffin recipe that you can put together ahead of time to simply grab and go. Pair a Chia Muffin, Make Ahead Zucchini Bread, or any other recipe lower in calories with a piece of fruit for more fiber or a low-fat yogurt for more protein to achieve the balance. These options blow your standard grab-and-go options — like a refined carb-filled bagel — out of the water with solid nutrition to start your day on a healthy foot in no time.

Whole-Wheat Banana French Toast

Prep time: 10 minutes • **Cook time:** 10–20 minutes • **Yield:** 4 servings

Ingredients	*Directions*
4 eggs (2 full, 2 egg whites)	*1* In a large bowl, whisk together two full eggs and two egg whites (discard two yolks), skim milk, and vanilla.
¾ cups skim milk	
½ teaspoon pure vanilla extract	*2* In a small bowl, mash up peeled bananas with a fork and add in nutmeg.
2 ripe bananas	
⅛ teaspoon nutmeg	*3* Lay out 4 slices of whole wheat bread and spread banana mixture on one side of each. Place other 4 slices on top to create a sandwich.
8 slices whole wheat bread	
2 tablespoons olive oil	*4* Dip each sandwich into the egg mixture so that entire sandwich is moistened.
	5 Heat 2 tablespoons olive oil in a large sauté pan over medium heat.
	6 Add bread sandwiches and cook on each side for about 5 minutes or until nicely browned.

Per serving: Calories 312; Fat 11 g; Saturated Fat 2g; Cholesterol 84mg; Sodium 350mg; Total Carbohydrate 39g; Dietary Fiber 5g; Protein 15g per sandwich.

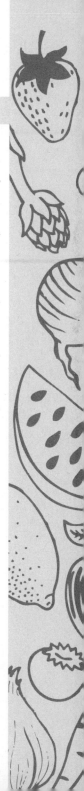

Oatmeal Peanut Butter Pancakes

Prep time: 10 minutes • **Cook Time:** 5 minutes • **Yield:** 1 serving

Ingredients	*Directions*
⅓ **cup rolled oats**	*1* In a food processor, pulse rolled oats until flour-like.
⅛ **cup whole wheat flour**	
½ **teaspoon baking soda**	*2* In a large bowl, combine ground oats, flour, baking soda, and cinnamon.
¾ **teaspoon cinnamon**	
2 egg whites	*3* In a separate bowl, whisk together egg whites with skim milk, maple syrup, and peanut butter.
½ **cup skim milk**	
1 teaspoon maple syrup	*4* Stir the wet ingredients in with the dry.
1 tablespoon all natural peanut butter	*5* Spray large skillet with olive oil spray and heat over medium heat.
Olive oil cooking spray	
	6 Pour about ¼ cup full of batter onto skillet in two or three pancakes, keep about 2 inches apart, and cook until you see bubbles. Flip and cook on other side for about 2 minutes or until browned.

Per serving: Calories 350; Fat 10g; Saturated Fat 1g; Cholesterol 2mg; Sodium 250mg; Carbohydrate 45g; Dietary Fiber 5g; Protein 20g for entire recipe.

Everyday Mixed Berry Parfait

Prep time: 5 minutes • **Yield:** 1 serving

Ingredients	Directions
6 ounces low-fat plain Greek yogurt	**1** Combine the yogurt, almonds, cereal, and berries in a large glass or bowl.
1 tablespoon sliced almonds	
2 tablespoons high fiber cereal	**2** Add stevia on top and enjoy!
1 cup mixed berries (blueberry, raspberry, strawberry)	
1 packet stevia	

Per serving: Calories 250; Fat 3.5g; Cholesterol 0mg; Sodium 85mg; Carbohydrates 27g; Dietary Fiber 7g; Protein 20g for one parfait.

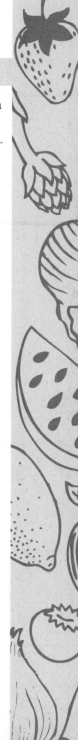

Ch-ch-ch-Chia Seed Muffin

Prep time: 15 minutes • **Cook time:** 20 minutes • **Yield:** 12 muffins

Ingredients

1 tablespoon ground chia seeds

1 ½ cups whole wheat flour

2 teaspoons baking soda

½ teaspoon salt

1 cup sweet potato puree or canned pumpkin

1 cup unsweetened apple sauce

2 egg whites

½ cup agave syrup

2 teaspoons lemon juice

1 teaspoon lemon zest

1 tablespoon pure vanilla extract

½ cup dried apples, chopped

Directions

1 Preheat oven to 350 F.

2 Mix together in a large bowl sweet potato puree, applesauce, egg whites, agave syrup, lemon juice, and vanilla.

3 Combine into the wet mixture chia seeds, whole wheat flour, baking soda, salt, lemon zest, and dried apples.

4 Scoop mixture into muffin pan until about ¾ full.

5 Bake for 15–20 minutes.

Per serving: Calories 140; Fat 0.5g; Sodium 300mg; Carbohydrates 32g; Fiber 2g; Protein 4g per muffin.

Apple, Cranberry, Pecan Energy Bars

Prep time: 15 minutes • **Cook time:** 20 minutes plus 10 minutes to cool • **Yield:** 8 bars

Ingredients	Directions
1 cup rolled oats	*1* Preheat oven to 350 F.
½ cup dried apples	*2* Line a 9×13 inch baking pan with parchment paper and spritz of cooking spray.
½ cup unsalted sunflower seeds	
½ cup toasted wheat germ	*3* Chop the rolled oats and dried apples in a food processor.
¼ cup whole wheat pastry flour	
½ cup dried cranberries	*4* Then add all remaining ingredients, except syrup and eggs, and pulse until mixture is finely chopped. Transfer this mixture into a large bowl.
½ cup unsalted pecans	
½ cup raisins	
½ cup powdered nonfat dry milk	*5* In a smaller bowl, beat the syrup and eggs. Add into the large bowl and stir until combined evenly.
½ teaspoon ground cinnamon	*6* Transfer mixture into baking pan and spread evenly.
½ teaspoon nutmeg	
⅓ cup pure maple syrup	*7* Bake for 20 minutes. Allow to cool for 10 minutes. Cut into 8 large squares.
2 large eggs	
Olive oil cooking spray	

Per serving: Calories 240; Fat 9g; Saturated Fat 1g; Cholesterol 47mg; Sodium 25mg; Carbohydrate 34g; Dietary Fiber 5g; Protein 8g per bar.

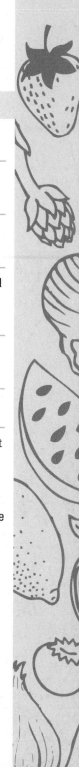

Make Ahead Zucchini Bread

Prep time: 10 minutes • **Cook time:** 50 minutes • **Yield:** 10 servings

Ingredients	Directions
2 egg whites	**1** Preheat oven to 350 degrees F.
½ cup brown sugar	
2 teaspoons vanilla extract	**2** Place egg whites in a large bowl. Add sugar and vanilla extract and blend well. Slowly add in vegetable oil.
2 teaspoons olive oil	
2 cups whole wheat flour	**3** In a separate bowl mix flour, baking soda, salt, baking powder, and cinnamon.
1 teaspoon salt	
1 teaspoon baking soda	**4** Combine bowl of dry ingredients with egg whites, sugar, and oil.
1 teaspoon cinnamon	
1 ½ cups shredded zucchini	**5** Alternate mixing wet ingredients into dry ingredients with zucchini and applesauce.
1 cup unsweetened applesauce	
1 cup chopped walnuts	**6** Add chopped walnuts.
	7 Grease Bundt pan with olive oil. (You can pour a tablespoon of olive oil on a paper towel and use to grease the pan.)
	8 Bake at 350 degrees F for about 50 minutes.

Per serving: Calories 225; Fat 9g; Saturated Fat 0.5; Cholesterol 0mg; Sodium 370mg; Carbohydrate 31g; Dietary Fiber 2.2g; Protein 7g per slice.

Greens, Eggs, and Cheese Burrito

Prep time: 20 minutes • **Cook time:** 10 minutes • **Yield:** 4 servings

Ingredients	*Directions*
2 teaspoons canola oil	**1** Heat the canola oil in nonstick skillet over medium-high heat.
¾ cup spinach, chopped	
1 bunch of scallions (3-5), chopped	**2** Cook scallions and spinach until softened.
1 cup black beans	**3** Add black beans and chili flakes and cook until beans are warmed through.
¼ teaspoon chili flakes	
8 eggs (use 4 full, 4 whites)	**4** Whisk together 4 full eggs and 4 egg whites and stir in cheese.
⅓ cup low-fat shredded cheese	
4 whole wheat tortillas	**5** Spray skillet with cooking spray and place on low heat. Add eggs and scramble until they are cooked through.
¼ cup salsa	
1 large tomato, seeded and diced	**6** Warm tortillas in microwave for 30 seconds each.
1 small avocado, cubed	**7** Spread salsa over each tortilla and then spoon black bean mixture, eggs, tomato, and avocado, favored to one side.
Olive oil cooking spray	
	8 Fold in corners of tortilla near edge where ingredients are heavier and roll up.

Per serving: Calories 400; Fat 18g; Saturated Fat 4g; Cholesterol 174mg; Sodium 500mg; Carbohydrate 38g; Dietary Fiber 10g; Protein 22g per burrito.

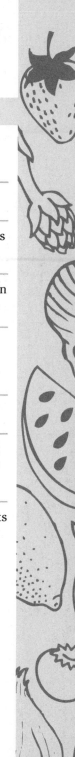

Rainbow Frittata & Fruit Salad

Prep time: 25 minutes • **Cook time:** 15 minutes • **Yield:** 4 servings

Ingredients	*Directions*
Frittata	**1** Whisk eggs and whites with turkey, skim milk in a medium bowl. Stir in feta cheese and basil and set aside.
6 eggs (3 whole, 3 whites only)	
4 ounces cooked lean ground turkey	**2** Put the cubed sweet potato into a glass measuring cup with 2 tablespoons of water and zap for 2–3 minutes to soften. Drain and set aside.
¼ cup skim milk	
¼ cup reduced fat feta cheese chunks	**3** Place olive oil in medium skillet over medium heat, add sweet potato, and cook for 4–5 minutes until browned.
2 tablespoons fresh basil, chopped	
¼ cup sweet potato, cubed	**4** Add red pepper, broccoli, tomato, and garlic to the skillet and cook on high heat for 2 minutes. Remove from heat and add to egg mixture in bowl.
1 tablespoon olive oil	
1 small red pepper, cut into strips	**5** Add a spritz of cooking spray to a clean skillet. Pour the recipe mixture onto the skillet and cook on low heat for 10 minutes. Broil for 1–3 minutes until browned.
½ cup broccoli florets	
¼ cup tomato, chopped	
1 small garlic clove, diced	**6** Let cool for 5–10 minutes. Combine all ingredients of fruit salad and put aside.
Olive oil cooking spray	
Fruit Salad	**7** Remove frittata from skillet by running a knife along the edges, flip onto a platter with fruit salad.
1 cup grapefruit, cubed	
½ cup strawberries, sliced	
½ cup blueberries	
1 cup apple, sliced	
1 cup low fat plain yogurt	
4 tablespoons ground flaxseed	

Per serving: Calories 325; Fat 13g; Saturated Fat 2g; Cholesterol 150mg; Sodium 300mg; Carbohydrate 25g; Dietary Fiber 6.5g; Protein 23g.

Strawberry, Banana, Cocoa Smoothie

Prep time: 5 minutes • **Yield:** 2 servings

Ingredients	*Directions*
1 banana	*1* Place all ingredients in blender and blend until smooth.
2 cups frozen strawberries	
1½ cup skim milk	
½ cup low fat yogurt	
1 tablespoon unsweetened dark cocoa powder	

Per serving: Calories 204; Fat 1.5g; Saturated Fat 1g; Cholesterol 6mg; Sodium 115mg; Carbohydrate 42g; Dietary Fiber 6g; Protein 10g per 8 ounce smoothie.

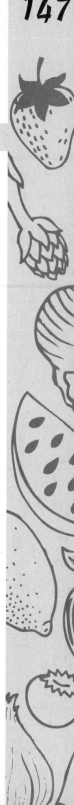

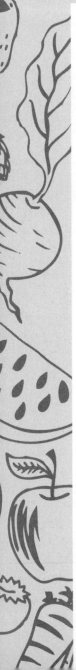

Energizing Citrus Ginger Smoothie

Prep time: 5 minutes • **Yield:** 1 serving

Ingredients	*Directions*
1 ½ cups low-fat plain Greek yogurt	*1* Place ingredients into blender and blend until smooth.
1 inch fresh ginger, peeled	
½ cup fresh orange chunks	
½ cup fresh pineapple chunks	
½ cup orange juice	
½ cup ice	

Per serving: Calories 300; Fat 5g; Saturated Fat 3g; Cholesterol 10mg; Sodium 70mg; Carbohydrate 45g; Dietary Fiber 4g; Protein 20g per 16 ounce smoothie.

Chapter 8

Powerful Lunches

In This Chapter

▶ Maximizing your midday meal to avoid that afternoon slump

▶ Understanding how packing your lunch can pack in an energy punch

*H*ow frequently do you go all day powered by coffee and snacks from a vending machine? Then it rolls around to 4 p.m. and you find yourself being unable to concentrate, without energy, and just ready for a hearty meal and bedtime. Although it may seem like skipping lunch saves you calories, it ultimately takes a toll on your metabolism. Without a lunch chock-full of nutrients, your blood sugar levels drop, you feel sluggish, and you tend to go overboard calorie-wise at dinnertime. Without lunch, the math never adds up to fewer calories or weight loss.

Planning ahead to have a lunch that powers you through the day doesn't have to be a chore. In this chapter, I provide simple recipes you can prep ahead of time and brown bag so that you keep your metabolism maximized throughout the day, no matter the situation. If you find yourself needing to take a lot of client or work lunch meetings, see Chapter 14 for best bets when dining out.

Salads, Soups, and Sandwiches

What constitutes a powerful lunch? It could be anything that has the balance you need of lean protein, complex carbs, and unsaturated fats — could be leftovers from dinner the night before, combinations of snacks, or even breakfast for lunch. But when I think of lunchtime, the standards are salads, soups, and sandwich options. They can be easily packed, refrigerated, and heated if necessary and give you all the nutrition you need to get through the day. They don't need to be boring either. With the recipes in this chapter for soup-er soups, satisfying salads, and better-for-you sandwiches, you'll get a variety of flavor combinations to keep your midday routine interesting.

Although salads, soups, and sandwiches might seem like innocuous dishes, put the wrong stuff in the bowl or between the bread, and you can have a calorie nightmare on your hands. Instead, be smart and keep in mind when prepping your powerful lunch:

- ✔ If you're not pairing your salad with a whole-wheat pita, you should include a complex carbohydrate with the meal, such as cut-up fruit, beans, and plenty of veggies besides lettuce.

- ✔ Make sure your sandwich bread isn't more calories than you've bargained for. Large wraps can count as 3–4 slices of bread, even if they're whole grains! Choose whole-wheat bread and refer to Chapter 5 for how to choose at the supermarket.

- ✔ Soups can be a meal as long as you've got veggies, beans, or another lean protein like white meat chicken in the mix. You may want to pair with a piece of fruit or have a small soup plus half a sandwich from the recipes in this chapter. A serving of soup like my White Bean Pumpkin can also make for a great winter snack.

Strawberry Fields of Kale

Yield: 1 Serving

Ingredients	Directions
Salad	**1** Mix together all dressing ingredients in a large bowl.
4 cups kale	
1 cup, halved strawberries	**2** Remove kale leaves from stems, wash, and break off small leaves. Add kale to the dressing bowl, mix, and massage with your hands thoroughly until leaves are covered.
7 walnut halves	
1 ounce avocado, cubed (about ⅕ medium avocado)	
Mustard Balsamic Dressing	**3** Add strawberries, walnuts, and avocado to the bowl and toss. Enjoy!
1 ounce Balsamic vinegar	
1 teaspoon Dijon mustard	
1 packet stevia	

Per serving: Calories 280; Fat 10g; Saturated Fat 1g; Sodium 175mg; Carbohydrate 31g; Dietary Fiber 9g; Protein 13g.

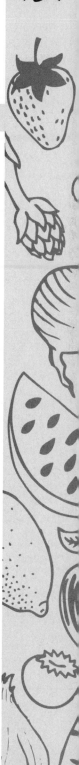

Chinese Chicken Salad

Prep time: 15 minutes • **Cook time:** 25 minutes • **Yield:** 4 servings

Ingredients	*Directions*
2 teaspoons toasted sesame oil	*1* Preheat oven to 350 degrees F.
1 pound skinless, boneless chicken breasts (about 3 large breasts)	*2* Brush sesame oil onto chicken breasts.
1 head Napa cabbage, thinly shredded	*3* Place chicken breasts on baking dish and bake for approximately 20–25 minutes. Once cooked, cut into ¼ inch slices.
1 bunch scallions, trimmed and thinly sliced	
¼ cup sliced almonds, toasted	*4* In bowl, mix Napa cabbage, carrot, scallions, sliced chicken, and almonds. Whisk together 1 tablespoon soy sauce, rice vinegar, garlic, ginger, oil, brown sugar, and chili sauce for the dressing and add to the salad.
1 large carrot, shredded	
1 tablespoon low-sodium soy sauce	
⅓ cup rice vinegar	
1 teaspoon minced garlic	
1 teaspoon minced ginger	
2 tablespoons canola oil	
2 tablespoons brown sugar	
1 ½ teaspoon chili sauce	

Per serving: Calories 317; Fat 15g; Saturated Fat 1.5g; Cholesterol 66mg; Sodium 475mg; Carbohydrate 12.5g; Dietary Fiber 3.5g; Protein 28g.

Turkey Taco Salad

Prep time: 10 minutes • **Cook time:** 10 minutes • **Yield:** 4 servings

Ingredients	*Directions*
2 tablespoons olive oil	*1* Heat 1 tablespoon olive oil in skillet over med-high heat.
¾ pound lean ground white turkey meat	
1 garlic clove, minced	*2* Add ground turkey, garlic, and chili powder until browned about 5–10 minutes. Remove from heat.
1 tablespoon chili powder	
1 cup cooked black beans	*3* In a large bowl mix black beans, tomatoes, 1 tablespoon olive oil, lime juice, and pepper.
4 medium tomatoes, diced	
2 tablespoons fresh lime juice	*4* Mix tomato and lime juice mixture with lettuce, cheddar cheese, and cooked turkey meat. Ole!
¼ teaspoon freshly ground black pepper	
2 hearts romaine lettuce, chopped	
½ cup low-fat cheddar cheese, shredded	

Per serving: Calories 405; Fat 14g; Saturated Fat 4g; Cholesterol 65mg; Sodium 150mg; Carbohydrates 37g; Dietary Fiber 10g; Protein 30g.

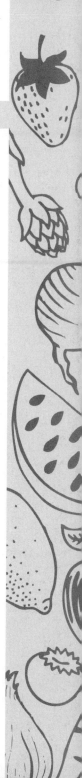

Quinoa Greek Salad

Prep time: 1 hour, 15 minutes • **Cook time:** 20 minutes • **Yield:** 4 servings

Ingredients	*Directions*
Greek Dressing	**1** Blend together lemon juice, vinegar, oregano, and garlic in a small bowl. Whisk in olive oil until emulsified.
3 tablespoons freshly squeezed lemon juice	
2 tablespoon red wine vinegar	**2** Heat quinoa in saucepan with 2 cups of water. Bring to boil and cook until quinoa has absorbed all the water, about 20 minutes.
¼ teaspoon dried oregano	
1 clove garlic, minced	
1 tablespoon olive oil	**3** Mix quinoa with tomatoes, onion, cucumber, feta cheese, olives, and dressing. Refrigerate for 1 hour.
Quinoa Salad	
1 cup quinoa	
1 medium red tomato, cubed	
1 red onion, thinly sliced	
1 cucumber, cubed	
½ cup part-skim feta cheese, crumbled	
½ cup kalamata olives	

Per serving: Calories 275; Fat 9g; Saturated Fat 1.5g; Cholesterol 5mg; Sodium 325mg; Carbohydrates 34g; Dietary Fiber 4.5g; Protein 10g.

White Bean Pumpkin Soup

Prep time: 10 minutes • **Cook time:** 15 minutes • **Yield:** 4 servings

Ingredients	*Directions*
½ **pound dried white cannellini beans**	**1** Cover the beans with water (at least 1 inch) and leave them in refrigerator overnight. Drain beans and put in food processor until they are pureed.
1 tablespoon olive oil	
1 onion, finely chopped	
2 15-ounce cans of pumpkin puree	**2** In a large saucepan sauté onions in olive oil until they are translucent. Add pumpkin puree, white bean puree, vegetable stock, pepper, garlic, and ginger and put heat on medium. Simmer for 5–10 minutes. Add milk and heat for an additional 5 minutes.
3 cups low-sodium vegetable stock	
½ **teaspoon freshly ground pepper**	
2 garlic cloves, minced	
½ **teaspoon ground ginger**	
1 cup 1% milk	

Per serving: Calories 202; Fat 4.5g; Saturated Fat 1.2g; Cholesterol 3mg; Sodium 231mg; Carbohydrates 33g; Dietary Fiber 11g; Protein 8g.

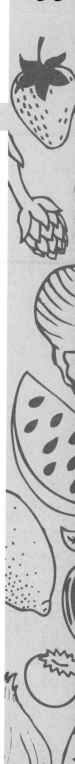

Hearty Lentil and Minestrone Soup

Prep time: 20 minutes • **Cook time:** 50 minutes • **Yield:** 8 servings

Ingredients	*Directions*
1 teaspoon olive oil	**1** Heat olive oil in a Dutch oven (large saucepan or stock-pot) over medium-high heat.
1 medium onion, finely chopped	
1 medium carrot, finely chopped	**2** Add onion, carrot, celery, cabbage, parsley, oregano, and garlic and sauté for 5 minutes.
1 stalk celery, chopped	
1 cup finely chopped cabbage	**3** Add water, salt, pepper, broth and bring to a boil. Add the remainder of ingredients (except spinach) and simmer for about 45 minutes. Stir in spinach. Remove from heat and enjoy!
2 tablespoons minced fresh parsley	
1 teaspoon dried oregano	
2 cloves of garlic, minced	
2 cups water	
¼ teaspoon salt	
¼ teaspoon freshly ground black pepper	
4 cups fat-free, low sodium chicken broth	
16 ounces lentils	
1 medium sweet potato, peeled and cubed	
½ cup pearl barley (uncooked)	
2 cups fresh spinach (or leafy green vegetable of your choosing)	

Per serving: Calories 285; Fat 1.5g; Sodium 385mg; Carbohydrates 50g; Dietary Fiber 20.7g; Protein 18g.

Salmon Bahn Mi Sandwich

Prep time: 35 minutes • **Cook time:** 25 minutes • **Yield:** 4 servings

Ingredients	*Directions*
Slaw	**1** Preheat oven to 375 degrees F.
¼ cup water	
¼ cup sugar	**2** To make slaw, combine water, sugar and vinegar in a saucepan, and bring to a boil. Remove from heat and cool. Add carrot and daikon, to slaw. Refrigerate for 30 minutes.
¼ cup distilled white vinegar	
½ cup julienned carrot	
½ cup julienned daikon radish	**3** Season salmon with olive oil, garlic powder, and pepper. Bake salmon in oven for 20 minutes or until crisp around the edges.
Seasoned Salmon	
6 ounce wild salmon	
1 teaspoon olive oil	**4** Slice baguettes lengthwise. Bake baguettes for about 5 minutes in oven. Cut salmon and put on baguettes. Add cilantro and cucumber slices to baguette. Top with slaw.
¼ teaspoon garlic powder	
Dash freshly ground pepper	
Sandwiches	
4 whole wheat baguettes	
½ cup fresh cilantro	
¼ medium cucumber, cut lengthwise into 4 slices	

Per serving: Calories 301; Fat 5.8g; Saturated Fat 0.7g; Cholesterol 30 mg; Sodium 350mg; Carbohydrates 49g; Dietary Fiber 7g; Protein 18g.

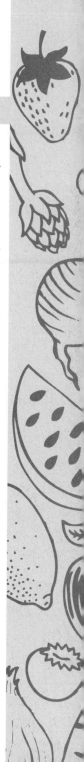

Veggie Burger Wrap Up

Prep time: 20 minutes • **Cook time:** 5–10 minutes • **Yield:** 6 servings

Ingredients	*Directions*
8 ounces shelled frozen edamame	*1* Boil edamame in water as directed by package. Drain and use potato masher to mash kidney beans and edamame in a bowl until slightly chunky.
8 ounces cooked kidney beans	
1 red onion, chopped	*2* Add onion, walnuts, carrots, bread crumbs, scallions, parsley, and soy sauce and season with pepper. Combine ingredients with hands. Form the bean mixture into 6 patties.
⅓ cup chopped walnut	
1 carrot, shredded	
1 cup whole wheat breadcrumbs	
2 scallions, finely chopped	*3* Heat olive oil in pan and add patties. Cook for 2–3 minutes on each side.
2 tablespoons chopped fresh parsley	
2 teaspoons low-sodium soy sauce	*4* Place 1 leaf lettuce and 1 tablespoon salsa on each tortilla. Add patty and wrap up!
Dash freshly ground pepper	
3 tablespoons olive oil	
4 whole wheat tortillas	
4 large leafs lettuce	
4 tablespoons salsa	

Per serving: Calories 402; Fat 12g; Saturated Fat 1g; Sodium 300mg; Carbohydrates 56g; Dietary Fiber 12.5g; Protein 19.5g.

Deli Style Tuna Salad Sandwich

Prep time: 15 minutes • **Yield:** 2 servings

Ingredients	Directions
½ teaspoon freshly ground pepper	**1** Combine all ingredients except the pita and spoon evenly into pita pockets.
½ small red onion, chopped finely	
1 celery stalk, chopped finely	
Pinch of dill	
2 tablespoons minced fresh parsley	
6-ounce pouch of chunk light tuna fish	
2 tablespoons low-fat mayonnaise	
2 whole wheat pita pockets	

Per serving: Calories 310; Fat 7.2g; Saturated Fat 0.8g; Cholesterol 49mg; Sodium 375mg; Carbohydrates 36g; Dietary Fiber 6.2g; Protein 28g.

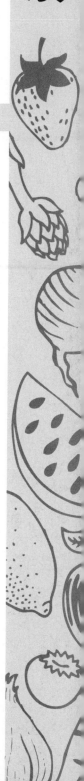

Chicken Artichoke Mini Melts

Prep time: 15 minutes • **Cook time:** 20 minutes • **Yield:** 4 servings

Ingredients	*Directions*
1 chicken breast, boneless and skinless	*1* Preheat oven to 400 degrees F.
Freshly ground pepper to taste	*2* Season chicken breast with pepper. Heat olive oil in medium skillet over med heat and cook chicken for 4–5 minutes per side. Cut chicken into small cubes.
2 tablespoons olive oil	
4 whole wheat English muffins	
2 tomatoes, seeded and chopped	*3* Lay English muffins on baking sheet. Place tomatoes, artichoke, cheese, and chicken on top of English muffins and bake for 10 minutes. Garnish with basil.
¼ cup artichoke, finely chopped	
¼ cup grated part-skim Parmesan cheese	
2 tablespoons fresh basil leaves	

Per serving: Calories 315; Fat 11g; Saturated Fat 2g; Cholesterol 42mg; Sodium 400mg; Carbohydrates 33.5g; Dietary Fiber 7.5g; Protein 22g.

Chapter 9

Delicious and Nutritious Dinners, Appetizers, and Sides

In This Chapter

▶ Whipping up recipes like a pro for a nutritious dinner

▶ Learning how to end your day on a metabolism-boosting high note

*E*nding the day with a light but nutritious dinner can help you finish getting all the nutrients you need while keeping your metabolism in high gear. Also, ensuring that you have a balance between complex carbohydrates and lean proteins, without foods high in saturated fat can help promote a good night's sleep. That way, you set yourself up for success for tomorrow.

When you have a hectic work and life schedule, making time for healthy dinner may be your biggest obstacle. You go to work, take your kids for after-school activities, or just have a busy day, and by the time you get home, it seems the easiest thing to do is to order delivery pizza or Chinese food. But this doesn't have to be the case. In this chapter, I provide easy dinner recipes that you can either prepare ahead and freeze or whip up the day of for a delicious dinner the entire family can enjoy.

Exploring Different Cuisines

Making a healthy dinner doesn't only have to mean grilled chicken and steamed vegetables or a salad with grilled fish on top. By being a bit adventurous with ingredients and testing the waters of different cuisines, your taste buds and metabolism will thank you.

Variety is key. Having the same meals over and over is boring, and you're less likely to stick to it in the long run. Mixing things up with a variety of flavors, spices, and nutrients helps keep your metabolism on a boosted path.

You may think you can only have Mexican food as a treat when out to eat, but there are ways to increase the nutrient density and healthfulness — try the Sirloin Tacos in this chapter. Similarly, you'll have recipes for Italian, Japanese, and Indian-inspired dishes to keep you satisfied, so that you're not craving the delivery menu.

If you're cooking for one, to save time and money, pick a theme for the week when it comes to cuisine. For example, if you buy whole wheat tortillas, low-fat shredded cheese, black beans, avocados, and corn, you can make a plethora of dishes throughout the week with these versatile ingredients.

Mixing and Matching

If you haven't gotten the memo yet, balancing your meal is the secret to metabolism-boosting success. When you just have carbohydrate, like pasta with tomato sauce, without an added source of protein, your metabolism doesn't have to work as hard to digest, your blood sugar levels spike, you aren't as satisfied, and you'll be craving another meal or snack soon after. Mix and match these recipes to meet your calorie needs for the meal.

Always pair carbohydrates with a serving of protein and heart-healthy fat. It doesn't matter whether you eat the foods directly together in a combo dish or separately as an appetizer or a side. For example, my Tofu Teriyaki is a lower-in-calorie protein dish, so pair with a grain and/or vegetable side for complex carbohydrates to complete the meal. Or simply serve with brown rice and a side salad. You can also combine lower-in-calorie dishes together, like Quinoa Stuffed Peppers with my Roasted Beet and Feta Salad, for a blend of flavors and nutrition.

Dishes like my Angel Hair with Shrimp and Snow Peas or Sirloin Tacos combine all the components of a balanced meal and can be eaten on its own. Same with vegetarian options like my mom's healthified Spinach Lasagna recipe. When in doubt of what to add to a meal like the Pistachio Crusted Chicken, so that you're more satisfied, you can never go wrong with leafy greens like Crunchy Kale to help fill you up with more fiber and get your veggie servings in for the day.

Pistachio Crusted Chicken with Mustard Sauce

Prep time: 10 minutes • **Cook time:** 40 minutes • **Yield:** 4 servings

Ingredients	Directions
Pistachio Crusted Chicken	_1_ Preheat oven to 400 degrees F. Spray a baking sheet with non-stick cooking spray and put aside.
¼ cup finely chopped pistachios	_2_ In a medium bowl, mix pistachios and whole wheat bread crumbs. In a separate small bowl, pour buttermilk, olive oil, and black pepper.
¼ cup whole wheat bread crumbs	
¼ cup low fat buttermilk	_3_ Cut each breast of chicken into two. Dip each piece in the wet mixture, then dip into the pistachio and breadcrumb mix to coat.
1 tablespoon olive oil	
black pepper, to taste	
2 large (about 12 ounces) skinless, boneless chicken breasts	_4_ Place on baking sheet and bake for about 30–40 minutes or until crust is browned.
Mustard Sauce	_5_ Mix together all mustard sauce ingredients.
½ cup Dijon mustard	_6_ Plate two pieces of chicken and drizzle about 2–3 tablespoons of sauce (or use to dip) for each serving.
1 tablespoon dry white wine	
1 tablespoon olive oil	
1 clove of garlic, minced	
1 tablespoon minced fresh or dried tarragon	
1 teaspoon minced and peeled fresh ginger	

Per serving: Calories 265; Fat 14g; Saturated Fat 2g; Cholesterol 50mg; Sodium 350mg; Carbohydrate 9g; Dietary Fiber 2.5g; Protein 22g.

Spinach Lasagna

Prep time: 15 minutes • **Cook time:** 1 hour 30 minutes • **Yield:** 6 servings

Ingredients	*Directions*
1 pound part skim ricotta cheese	*1* Preheat oven to 350 degrees.
1 ½ cups shredded part skim mozzarella	*2* In a large bowl, mix ricotta, 1 cup of mozzarella, spinach, oregano, and pepper.
1 10-ounce package frozen spinach, thawed and drained	*3* Spray a lasagna pan and layer ⅓ of the tomato sauce, ½ lasagna noodles, and about ½ cheese mixture. Again, sauce, noodles, and cheese mixture. Last layer is the remaining tomato sauce and top with remaining mozzarella.
¾ teaspoon oregano	
⅛ teaspoon pepper	
1 large jar (24 ounces) low-sodium tomato sauce	
1 package no boil, whole-wheat lasagna noodles	*4* Pour 1 cup of water around perimeter of pan and cover tightly with aluminum foil.
1 cup water	*5* Bake at 350 degrees for 1 hour and 15 minutes or until bubbly.
	6 Take out and pull back aluminum foil. Let cool for 10 minutes before eating.

Per serving: Calories 355; Fat 15g; Saturated Fat 5g; Cholesterol 39mg; Sodium 450mg; Carbohydrate 40g; Dietary Fiber 7g; Protein 23g.

Sirloin Tacos with Guacamole

Prep time: 20 minutes • **Cook time:** 15 minutes • **Yield:** 5 servings

Ingredients	*Directions*
Sirloin Tacos	*1* Mix ½ cup lime juice, olive oil, chili powder, and black pepper in a bowl. Baste sirloin with mixture and place on skillet.
¼ **cup fresh lime juice (about 2 limes)**	
2 tablespoons olive oil	*2* Cook sirloin on high for about 5 minutes on each side. Cut into 1 inch strips.
½ **tablespoon chili powder**	
½ **tablespoon black pepper**	*3* Scoop avocado and all ingredients for guacamole and pico de gallo mix into bowl. Mash with a fork until well combined.
1 pounds lean sirloin steak	
10 whole wheat tortillas taco-size	
Guacamole and Pico de Gallo mix	*4* Grill tortillas to warm up for 30 seconds on each side.
1 ½ ripe avocados	*5* Evenly spread sirloin and guacamole mix among the tortillas.
½ **small red onion, diced**	
¼ **cup diced tomatoes**	
½ **cup diced green or red pepper**	
¼ **cup chopped fresh cilantro**	
1 tablespoon fresh lime juice	

Per serving (2 soft tacos): Calories 620; Fat 25g; Saturated Fat 4g; Cholesterol 81mg; Sodium 400mg; Carbohydrates 60g; Dietary Fiber 13g; Protein 39g.

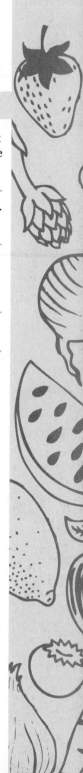

Blackened Cajun Salmon with Mango Salsa

Prep time: 15 minutes • **Cook time:** 10 minutes • **Yield:** 4 servings

Ingredients	Directions

Salmon

4 salmon steaks (about 1 pound)

1 teaspoon white pepper

1 teaspoon garlic powder

1 teaspoon turmeric

1 teaspoon cayenne pepper

1 teaspoon paprika

1 teaspoon olive oil

Salsa

2 large ripe mangos, peeled and chopped

1 red bell pepper, diced

1 small red onion, chopped

1 tablespoon finely chopped jalapeno

2 tablespoons chopped cilantro

¼ cup lime juice

4 small mint leaves

1 Combine all salsa ingredients in a large bowl and cover with Saran wrap. Refrigerate to allow flavors to mix.

2 Combine salmon seasonings in a small bowl and rub the mixture on the salmon fillets.

3 Heat olive oil in a skillet on medium heat and add salmon.

4 Starting with skin side up, cook for about 5 minutes on each side or until blackened and salmon flakes easily.

5 Top with mango salsa and enjoy.

Per serving: Calories 336; Fat 14; Saturated Fat 2.5g; Cholesterol 71mg; Sodium 70mg; Carbohydrates 21g; Dietary Fiber 3.5g; Protein 26g.

Spaghetti Squash with Pine Nuts, Tomato, and Chickpeas

Prep time: 15 minutes • **Cook time:** 45 minutes • **Yield:** 4 servings

Ingredients	Directions
1 medium (about 4.5 pounds) spaghetti squash, halved	*1* Preheat oven to 450 degrees F. Cover an oven tray with aluminum foil.
3 tablespoons olive oil	
Dash of ground black pepper	*2* Scrape out seeds from squash. Season spaghetti squash with 2 tablespoons olive oil and ground black pepper. Put the squash face down on tray and roast for 30–40 minutes. Remove from oven, let cool, and scrape squash with fork.
1 cup crushed tomatoes, canned or jarred	
1 garlic clove, finely chopped	
¼ cup pine nuts	*3* In skillet heat crushed tomatoes, 1 tablespoon olive oil, garlic, pine nuts, and chickpeas.
¼ cup cooked chickpeas	
	4 Toss spaghetti squash with crushed tomato sauce and enjoy!

Per serving: Calories 354; Fat 15g; Saturated Fat 2g; Sodium 300mg; Carbohydrate 41.5g; Dietary Fiber 12.5g; Protein 14g.

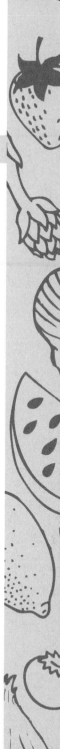

Spicy Vegetarian Chili

Prep time: 20 minutes • **Cook time:** 25 minutes • **Yield:** 6 servings

Ingredients	*Directions*
1 large onion, chopped	*1* In large pot, sauté onion, green pepper, red pepper, carrots, jalapeno, and garlic with olive oil for about 5 minutes.
1 large green pepper, chopped	
1 large red pepper, chopped	
3 medium carrots, chopped	*2* Add vegetable broth, tomatoes, kidney beans, and black beans. Mix well.
1 jalapeno, chopped	
6 cloves garlic, minced	*3* Then add in seasonings and cook over medium heat for 20 minutes.
2 tablespoons olive oil	
1 cup low sodium vegetable broth	
1 32-ounces crushed tomatoes, canned or jarred	
1 cup cooked kidney beans	
1 cup cooked black beans	
2 tablespoons chili powder	
1 tablespoon ground cumin	
2 teaspoons ground coriander	
1 tablespoon hot pepper sauce	

Per serving: Calories 365; Fat 6g; Saturated Fat 1g; Sodium 250mg; Carbohydrates 62g; Dietary Fiber 17g; Protein 19g.

Angel Hair with Shrimp and Snow Peas

Prep time: 15 minutes • **Cook time:** 20 minutes • **Yield:** 6 servings

Ingredients	*Directions*
2 pounds shrimp, peeled and deveined	*1* Preheat oven to 400 degrees F.
5 tablespoons olive oil	*2* Place shrimp on a baking sheet. Combine 1 table-spoon of olive oil with ½ teaspoon pepper and brush over shrimps. Roast for 6–8 minutes.
½ teaspoon pepper	
1 pound whole wheat angel hair pasta	*3* Place snow peas, cherry tomatoes, and asparagus on separate baking sheet and drizzle with 1 tablespoon of olive oil. Bake for about 10 minutes.
1 lemon, zested and juiced	
½ cup snow peas	
½ cup cherry tomatoes, halved	*4* Boil angel hair pasta in large pot and cook for about 3 minutes. Drain the pasta and save about ½ cup of cooking water.
1 pound asparagus, cut into 2-inch pieces	
	5 Toss pasta with 3 tablespoons olive oil, lemon zest, and juice and ½ cup of reserved cooking water. Split among plates and distribute snow peas, cherry toma-toes, asparagus, and shrimp evenly to each serving.

Per serving: Calories 526; Fat 14.7g; Saturated Fat 2g; Cholesterol 295mg; Sodium 350mg; Carbohydrate 50g; Dietary Fiber 10g; Protein 35g.

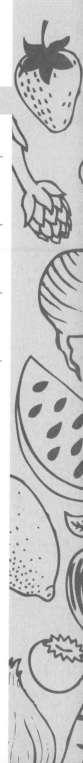

Quinoa Stuffed Peppers

Prep time: 15 minutes • **Cook time:** 1 hour and 15 minutes • **Yield:** 6 servings

Ingredients	*Directions*
3 tablespoons olive oil	*1* Preheat oven to 400 degrees F.
2 large shallots, diced	
2 zucchinis, grated	*2* Heat 2 tablespoons of olive oil in a large saucepan and add shallots, zucchini, cumin, salt, and pepper. Cook for about 5 minutes.
½ tablespoon ground cumin	
1 teaspoon salt	
1 teaspoon freshly ground black pepper	*3* Add 1 more tablespoon olive oil to the saucepan. Add quinoa and cook for about 2 minutes. Add white wine and cook until wine has evaporated. Then add 1 ½ cups of water and bring to a boil. Cover pan and simmer until all the water has been absorbed, about 5 minutes.
1 ½ cups quinoa	
¼ cup white wine	
6 red or yellow bell peppers	*4* Cut the top off the peppers and remove all seeds and ribs. Place peppers in baking dish and spoon quinoa mixture into peppers. Fill the baking dish with ¾ inch hot water and bake for about 50–60 minutes.
½ cup shredded low-fat mozzarella cheese	
	5 Sprinkle cheese and broil for 2 minutes on medium.

Per serving: Calories 286; Fat 11g; Saturated Fat 2g; Sodium 445mg; Carbohydrates 36g; Dietary Fiber 6g; Protein 10g.

Tofu Teriyaki

Prep time: 10 minutes • **Cook time:** 45 minutes • **Yield:** 6 servings

Ingredients	*Directions*
¼ cup low-sodium soy sauce	*1* Heat broiler to high.
1 tablespoon stevia	
2 tablespoons dry sherry	*2* Combine soy sauce, stevia, dry sherry, rice vinegar, garlic, ginger, and red pepper flakes and stir well.
2 tablespoons rice vinegar	
2 garlic cloves, minced	
1 teaspoon finely grated fresh ginger	*3* Mix tofu with sauce and spread on broiler pan. Broil for 15 minutes on each side. Flip once more and cook for another 5–10 minutes.
¼ teaspoon red pepper flakes	*4* Sprinkle with sesame seeds and broil for 1 more minute. Enjoy!
2 16-oz containers of firm or extra-firm tofu, cubed	
2 teaspoons sesame seeds	

Per serving: Calories 210; Fat 11g; Saturated Fat 2g; Sodium 600mg; Carbohydrates 4g; Fiber 1.5g; Protein 13g.

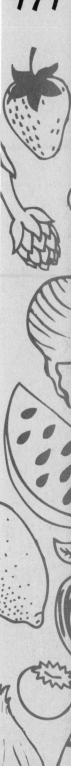

Crunchy Kale and Brussels Sprouts

Prep time: 5 minutes • **Cook time:** 45 minutes • **Yield:** 4 servings

Ingredients	*Directions*
2 bunches of kale	*1* Preheat over to 300 degrees F.
1 cup quartered Brussels sprouts	*2* Tear off leaves from bunches of kale. Put leaves in bowl with Brussels sprouts.
2 tablespoons olive oil	
Ground black pepper	*3* Drizzle with olive oil, black pepper to taste, and mix well. Spread mixture evenly onto oven tray and bake for 30–45 minutes. Remove and let cool before eating.

Per serving: Calories 105; Fat 7.5g; Saturated Fat 1.1g; Sodium 34mg; Carbohydrates 9g; Dietary Fiber 2g; Protein 3g.

Chili Garlic Edamame

Prep time: 5 minutes • **Cook time:** 10 minutes • **Yield:** 4 servings

Ingredients	*Directions*
1 pound frozen edamame ½ tablespoon olive oil	**1** Boil edamame according to package. Drain and place in bowl and toss with chili powder.
¼ teaspoon red pepper flakes ½ teaspoon chili powder	**2** Heat olive oil, red pepper flakes, and minced garlic in a skillet. Toss in edamame and cook for 2–3 minutes.
2 garlic cloves, minced	**3** Remove from heat and add additional spice to taste.

Per serving: Calories 170; Fat 5g; Saturated Fat 0.5g; Sodium 23mg, Carbohydrate 17.1mg; Dietary Fiber 11.5g; Protein 14g.

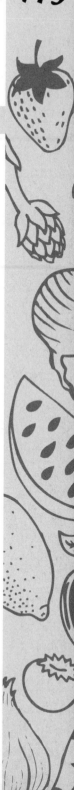

Roasted Beet and Feta Salad

Prep time: 10 minutes • **Cook time:** 45 minutes • **Yield:** 6 servings

Ingredients	*Directions*
6 large beets	*1* Preheat oven to 375 degrees F.
2 cups baby arugula	
1 large Asian pear, diced	*2* Cut off beet tops and thoroughly wash and dry beets. Wrap each in aluminum foil.
¼ cup crumbled feta cheese	
3 tablespoons extra virgin olive oil	*3* Place beets on oven tray and roast for about 45 minutes or until knife meets no resistance when sliced through the beet.
Freshly ground black pepper	
	4 Remove from oven and let cool. Peel beets and slice into ½-inch thick slices.
	5 Evenly spread arugula and diced pear among plates. Place beets on top of baby arugula and sprinkle feta cheese, drizzle olive oil, pepper to taste.

Per serving: Calories 120; Fat 8.5g; Saturated Fat 2g; Cholesterol 6mg; Sodium 110mg; Carbohydrates 11g; Dietary Fiber 2.2g; Protein 2g.

Mashed Sweet Potato and Butternut Squash

Prep time: 15 minutes • **Cook time:** 45 minutes • **Yield:** 6 servings

Ingredients	Directions
1 butternut squash (about 2 pounds)	**1** Cut the butternut squash in half lengthwise and remove seeds. Peel and cut sweet potatoes in half lengthwise. Place squash and sweet potatoes, cut side up on a foil-lined oven tray.
2 large sweet potato	
3 tablespoons olive oil	**2** In a saucepan, heat olive oil over low heat and whisk in stevia and ginger. Take off from heat.
1 packet stevia	
2 teaspoons ground ginger	
2 teaspoons cinnamon	**3** Brush the olive oil mixture onto the cut sides of the squash and potato. Sprinkle cinnamon on top.
½ cup raisins	
	4 Roast the squash and potatoes for about 45 minutes. Scoop out flesh of squash in a bowl. Cut up sweet potato in cubes and mash both together with fork.
	5 Add raisins and combine evenly.

Per serving: Calories 180; Fat 7g; Saturated Fat 1g; Sodium 25mg; Carbohydrate 30g; Dietary Fiber 4g; Protein 2g.

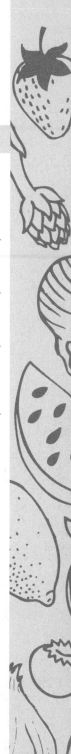

Bulgur Pilaf with Wild Mushrooms

Prep time: 30 minutes • **Cook time:** 20 minutes • **Yield:** 6 servings

Ingredients	*Directions*
2 cups water	*1* Boil water and add dried mushrooms. Allow mushrooms to plump, about 20 minutes. Strain the now mushroom stock and chop up any large mushrooms finely.
1 cup dried mushrooms	
2 tablespoons olive oil	
4 cups sliced fresh mushrooms of your choice like crimini, porcini, chantarelle	*2* In a large pan, heat 1 tablespoon olive oil. Add fresh mushrooms and cook until browned, about 20 minutes. Remove sliced mushrooms from pan and put aside.
1 small carrot, finely chopped	
1 ½ cups bulgur	*3* In same pan, add 1 tablespoon olive oil, carrot, and bulgur. Stir in chopped up mushrooms, mushroom stock, and broth. Bring to a boil and then simmer until broth has been absorbed by bulgur.
1 cup low sodium chicken broth	
2 tablespoons chopped fresh thyme	*4* Stir in sliced mushrooms, thyme, pepper, and chopped parsley. Serve hot or cold.
½ teaspoon fresh ground pepper	
2 tablespoons chopped parsley	

Per serving: Calories 182; Fat 5.4g; Saturated Fat 0.8g; Sodium 30mg; Carbohydrates 30mg; Dietary Fiber 7.7g; Protein 6.6g.

Chapter 10

Desserts and Snacks

In This Chapter

▶ Dispelling the belief that all snacks and desserts do you harm

▶ Understanding how to prepare healthful treats so you don't feel deprived

*I*f you ask me the number one reason why most "diets" fail, it's gotta be deprivation. When you start trying to eat healthier, you will inevitably cut foods from your daily routine — which then makes you constantly think about food and feel hungry, fatigued, and emotionally unsatisfied.

Typically, the items you cut out from what you eat on a fad diet are sweets and snack foods. But these foods aren't all "bad" (Chapter 4 can help you understand why you shouldn't think about food in terms of good and bad). A major part of the boosting-your-metabolism way is substituting the foods you eat with more nutritionally dense foods so that you're satisfied and energized throughout the day.

Smart Snacks

Note that *snack* is not a four-letter word. People who snack smart are more likely to lose weight and keep it off. Why?

✔ Snacks help keep your metabolism working during long stretches between meals.

✔ Having a snack can help keep you fueled throughout the day.

✔ A snack with complex carbs and lean protein can help prevent you from going into your next meal too ravenous.

When should you have a snack?

- ✔ You should snack only if you have a stretch of more than four hours between meals.

- ✔ The best time to snack is typically mid-afternoon, between lunch and dinner.

- ✔ Research shows that people who snack in the morning are more likely to weigh more. This is probably because they're snacking when they don't truly need it. Usually, there aren't many hours between breakfast and lunch on a workday. However, everyone has a different schedule — which is why in Chapter 6, my sample meal plans provide variable time tables for meals and snacks.

What should you snack on? Try the delicious and nutritious recipes in this section for snacks that are satisfying to your stomach and taste buds.

Guilt-Free Desserts

I love sweets. My day isn't complete without ice cream or chocolate. However, I stick to ½ to 1 cup ice cream or 1 ounce chocolate and choose only one or the other, once per day. When it comes to dessert, you may never think you're able to have it in moderation. But if you make concessions with your portions, how frequently you have dessert, or prep recipes that are a healthified versions of your favorites (which you may find in this chapter), you can certainly satisfy your sweet tooth, guilt-free.

In fact, I *encourage* you have dessert or another type of "fun food" once per day. If you absolutely love a food and completely *avoid* it, you're more likely to crave and overeat when faced with it.

Choco-Cinnamon Pudding

Prep time: <5 minutes • **Cook time:** 5 minutes • **Yield:** 4 servings

Ingredients	Directions
¼ cup cornstarch 2 tbsp sugar 3 tablespoons unsweetened cocoa 1 teaspoon cinnamon 1 ounce dark chocolate, cut into small pieces 2½ cups fat-free milk	**1** In a saucepan over medium heat, put in all the ingredients except the milk. **2** Gradually add the milk while stirring constantly. Stir until mixture comes to a boil. Boil for one minute and continue to stir. **3** Remove from heat and let cool or refrigerate before eating.

Per serving: Calories 156; Fat 2.8g; Cholesterol 5mg; Sodium 72mg; Carbohydrates 28g; Dietary Fiber 2g; Protein 6.5g.

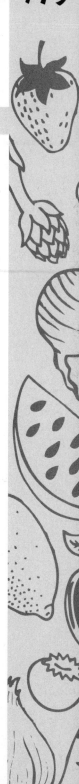

Banana Walnut "Ice Cream"

Prep time: 15 minutes • **Freeze time:** 1 hour • **Yield:** 1 serving

Ingredients	*Directions*
1 large banana, cut into small pieces	**1** Lay peeled banana pieces on a dish and freeze for 1–2 hours.
1 tablespoon dark chocolate chips	**2** While freezing, add chocolate chips and walnuts to mini chopper for chopping into smaller pieces. Remove and hold separately.
1 tablespoon chopped walnuts	**3** Once frozen, blend the banana, occasionally scraping down the sides of the blender. Blend until an ice cream-like consistency is reached.
	4 Add the chopped ingredients back in the blender and blend to incorporate into the ice cream, or just sprinkle them on top as a topping.

Per serving: Calories 203; Fat 7.3g; Saturated Fat 1.8g; Sodium 1 mg; Carbohydrates 37g; Dietary Fiber 4g; Protein 3g.

Coconut Cranberry Cookies

Prep time: 15 minutes • **Cook time:** 10 minutes • **Yield:** 40 cookies

Ingredients	*Directions*
2 cups whole-wheat flour	*1* Preheat oven to 350.
1 teaspoon baking soda	
½ cup vegetable oil	*2* Spread coconut in a thin layer on cookie sheet. Toast for 10 minutes. Increase oven to 375.
½ cup fat-free vanilla yogurt	
1½ cup agave syrup	*3* Whisk together flour and baking soda in a bowl. With an electric mixer mix oil, yogurt, and syrup until fluffy. Add flaxseed and stir. Fold in toasted coconut and cranberries.
1 tablespoon ground flaxseed	
1 cup sweetened shredded coconut	
1 cup dried cranberries	*4* Take 1 tablespoon of mixture and place on ungreased cookie sheet. Bake for 8–10 minutes.

Per Serving (1 cookie): Calories 105; Fat 3.5g; Saturated Fat 1.4g; Sodium 44mg; Carbohydrates 15g; Dietary Fiber 0.5g; Protein 1g.

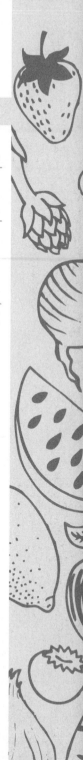

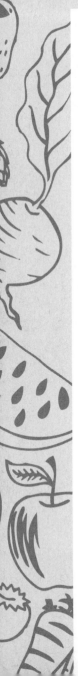

Green Tea Frozen Greek Yogurt

Prep time: 15 minutes • **Freeze time:** 1.5 hours • **Yield:** 1 serving

Ingredients	*Directions*
6 ounces fat free plain Greek-style yogurt	*1* Whisk yogurt with green tea powder and honey in a small bowl. Freeze for 30 minutes.
1 tablespoon Matcha Green tea powder	
2 teaspoons honey	*2* Remove bowl from freezer and whisk to break up frozen chunks. Mix in cherries and pomegranate seeds and return to freezer for 30 minutes. Remove and mash up and put back in freezer for another 30 minutes. Repeat.
¼ cup pitted cherries, halved	
1 tablespoon pomegranate seeds (alternatively use chopped nuts)	*3* Finally, remove mixture from freezer and blend with hand mixer until creamy.

Per serving: Calories 220; Fat 0g; Sodium 74mg; Carbohydrate 37g; Dietary Fiber 1.5g; Protein 17.5g.

Note: Make multiple servings ahead of time, freeze, and remove 10–15 minutes before eating.

Apple Pie Crumble

Prep time: 15 minutes • **Cook time:** 45 minutes • **Yield:** 6 servings

Ingredients	Directions
5 cups sliced and peeled apples like Fuji	*1* Preheat oven to 375 F.
3 tablespoons apple butter	*2* Combine apples and apple butter in a baking dish.
¼ cup whole wheat flour	
¼ cup oats, uncooked	*3* In a large bowl, mix flour, oats, sugar, cinnamon, margarine, and flaxseed until evenly combined. Add mixture to top of apples.
¼ cup packed light brown sugar	
1 teaspoon ground cinnamon	
3 tablespoons trans fat free margarine	*4* Bake for 45 minutes or until browned.
2 tablespoons ground flaxseed	

Per serving: Calories 136; Fat 1.4 g; Saturated Fat 0g; Sodium 95mg; Carbohydrates 30g; Dietary Fiber 3g; Protein 2g.

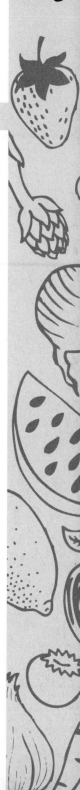

Frozen Yogurt Covered Blueberry Bites

Prep time: 5 minutes • **Freeze time:** 30 minutes–1 hour • **Yield:** 2 servings

Ingredients	Directions
½ pint fresh blueberries	**1** Line a baking sheet with wax paper.
6-ounce container nonfat vanilla Greek-style yogurt	**2** Using a toothpick, pick up one blueberry at a time and dip into yogurt until covered.
	3 Place on sheet and freeze bites for 30 minutes to an hour.

Per serving: Calories 121; Fat 0.5g; Sodium 39mg; Carbohydrates 21.5g; Dietary Fiber 2.5g; Protein 9g.

Sweet Potato Crisps

Prep time: 5 minutes • **Cook time:** 30 minutes • **Yield:** 4 servings

Ingredients	Directions
1 large sweet potato	**1** Preheat oven to 375 F.
1 tablespoon olive oil	**2** Cut sweet potato into thin slices or strips. Toss with olive oil and add your favorite herb or spice.
1 tablespoon chili powder (or your favorite herb or spice)	**3** Bake until crisp about 30 minutes.

Per serving: Calories 76; Fat 4g; Saturated Fat 0.5g; Sodium 35mg; Carbohydrate 10g; Dietary Fiber 2.1g; Protein 1.1g.

Popcorn Snack Bars

Prep time: 15 minutes • **Refrigerate time:** 1–2 hours • **Yield:** 6 servings

Ingredients	Directions
1 cup old-fashioned oats **½ cup almonds, sliced** **4 cups air-popped popcorn** **½ cup raisins** **½ cup honey**	**1** Preheat oven to 350. Line a shallow baking pan or sheet with parchment paper.
	2 Spread oats and almonds in one layer across the pan and bake for 10-15 minutes until golden.
	3 In a large bowl, mix up all the ingredients including the toasted almonds and oats.
	4 Spray a 9×13 pan with cooking spray and place the mixture in the pan. Use your hands to press down firmly. Spray your hands with cooking spray to help prevent sticking.
	5 Place in refrigerator for 1–2 hours. Remove and cut up into bars or pieces.

Per serving: Calories 195; Fat 5.2g; Saturated Fat 0.5g; Sodium 2mg; Carbohydrate 36g; Dietary Fiber 4g; Protein 4.5g.

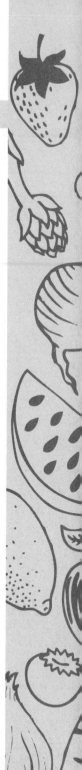

Spiced Chickpeas

Prep time: 5 minutes • **Cook time:** 30 minutes • **Yield:** 8 servings

Ingredients	*Directions*
2 cups cooked chickpeas 1 tablespoon olive oil	*1* Preheat oven to 450 F. Line a baking sheet with parchment paper.
2 teaspoons ground cumin 1 teaspoon chili powder	*2* Combine spices and oil in a small bowl. Add chickpeas to coat.
	3 Lay chickpeas on the baking sheet. Bake for 30 minutes, regularly turning with a spoon until crispy. Let cool for 20 minutes before eating.

Per serving: Calories 200; Fat 4.9g; Saturated Fat 0.5g; Sodium 16mg; Carbohydrates 30.7g; Dietary Fiber 9g; Protein 9.8g.

Part IV
Health and Lifestyle Issues

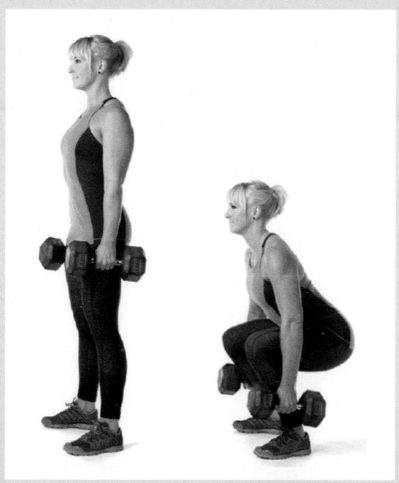

Photo by Bob McNamara

Old habits die hard, but remember they didn't develop overnight. It's easy to get frustrated and give up on healthy habits if you don't see results as quickly as you'd like. But remember, it's a lifestyle change, not a quick fix. Check out a free online article of mine that provides a wealth of tips and advice on how to really make some changes that will set you up in the long term (in fact, it used to be a chapter but we couldn't fit it into the book!). Find it at www.dummies.com/extras/boostingyourmetabolism/.

In this part . . .

✔ Stay active to boost your metabolism with great workouts, many of which you can do anywhere, anytime.

✔ Know how hormone-disrupting conditions can affect your metabolism — and what you can do about them.

✔ Get your household, family, and friends on board to keep you motivated and on track.

✔ Eat on-the-go at parties and restaurants without wrecking your metabolism achievements.

Chapter 11

Metabolism Workouts

• •

• •

This may surprise you, but I hear more excuses from clients about why they don't exercise than about why they're not making healthy changes in their diet. If you've had difficulty sticking to an exercise routine, you're not alone. When the weather gets cold or your life is hectic, you can stop being active, but you can never completely stop eating.

Although you may not have been blessed with an inherently fast metabolism, exercising is one of the major steps you can take to change the hand you've been dealt. Finding a routine that'll fit into your lifestyle no matter what isn't out of reach. I'm not *only* talking about burning more calories and building muscle. Calories aside, exercise improves your strength and confidence, and helps your mood, energy, and sleeping habits — which are all integral to a boosted metabolic rate.

This chapter teaches you how to work out both your body and your mind. Motivation comes from a place deep within yourself and is tied into being knowledgeable about what you can accomplish and how you'll get there. You'll learn to stop making excuses and start making changes with detailed routines for any fitness level. Then, by tracking your progress and how far you've gone literally and figuratively, exercise can become just another part of your daily routine.

Basics of Burning

Everyone carries excess fat differently, and it may seem like when you eat a doughnut, it goes straight to your thighs (or belly or buttocks). But it's not just the fat you eat that gets stored; anything you eat in excess of your need for fuel gets puts away by your body for later use like you're going into hibernation for the winter. When you get regular activity, you can burn off those excess calories so you don't store them as fat.

No matter where you store fat, you can rev up your burning furnace with activity. Consistent activity — especially weight-bearing, resistance exercises during which you build and tone muscle — can help offset the 5–10 percent in muscle mass decline per decade of life. That's one of the reasons your metabolism slows as you age. So you can give yourself a little wiggle room with your daily calorie intake by burning off more through exercise and building lean muscle mass.

The amount of calories muscle burns at rest is under contention. There are reports that say anywhere from 6–100 calories per pound, but personally I think it's more towards the low end: 5–20 calories per pound. Fat, by the way, burns about 2 calories per pound at rest.

So, why all the emphasis on building muscle? Because in the process, you're getting activity, burning more calories during and directly after every workout. Also, if you work on your muscle, your body will be more likely to release fat from your least favorite body part, as long as you're keeping up with the calorie deficit.

During the act

I'm sure you've heard of the "Fat Burning Zone" or at least seen the graphic for one on your treadmill, elliptical, or stationary bicycle. The truth is that your body is always using both fat and carbohydrate for energy, just in different ratios, depending on the type and intensity of exercise you're doing.

The intensity of your exercise is defined by how fast your heart is beating and at what percentage of your maximum heart rate. Your maximum heart rate equals 220 minus your age in years. For example, if you're 50 years old, your maximum heart rate is 170 beats per minute.

Many exercise machines can monitor your heart rate through sensors that you touch. Otherwise, to determine what level of exercise you're at, you can take your heart rate manually. Stop briefly during your workout and take your pulse using the tips of your index and middle fingers on your wrist. Count how many beats you feel for 30 seconds and multiply by 2 to get your beats per minute.

Here are the levels of exercise as I see them:

- ✓ **Couch potato:** While you're sitting there reading this book, your body is burning calories off at a ratio of about 50 percent carbohydrate and 50 percent fat.

- ✓ **Quick burst:** If you sat up and started sprinting, the carbohydrate percentage would go up, because it's more easily broken down and accessible to muscles.

This type of quick-burst exercise, lasting up to about two minutes, is also known as *anaerobic* exercise, meaning your body doesn't use as much oxygen to perform it as it would for more prolonged activity. Anaerobic exercise produces lactic acid, a compound that can build up in the blood and cause fatigue. Over time, you become more and more able to tolerate this lactic acid, which prolongs the time before your muscles tire, improving your endurance. After exercise, your body needs to take in more oxygen to break down this lactic acid, burning calories after the act.

✔ **Moderate intensity:** Over time, when you're engaging in moderate-intensity exercise, like walking briskly, you're in "fat-burning" mode. A higher percentage of calories that you burn are from fat because your body isn't working too hard, so it has the resources to break down fat, which is harder to access. In this mode, your heart rate is about 50–70 percent of your maximum rate.

✔ **High intensity:** When your heart rate hits 70–85 percent of your maximum, your body goes back to using more carbohydrates because it needs the energy more rapidly.

Maybe it's surprising to you that your body is burning a higher percentage calories from fat at a lower intensity, but that doesn't translate into more fat calories burned overall. Athletes aren't lean because they focus on the percentage of time they're in the fat-burning zone. They're lean because they work out harder and longer and burn more calories overall. Table 11-1 shows an example of what you burn at different intensities for the same amount of time.

Table 11-1	Low-Intensity versus High-Intensity Workout Results*		
Activity (30 min)	*Total Calories Burned*	*Fat Percentage*	*Fat Calories Burned*
Reading	45	50	22.5
Walking (3.0 m.p.h.)	160	65	104
Running (7.5 m.p.h.)	450	40	180

* Based on a person who weighs 160 pounds

Don't only track your progress by weight loss because when you build muscle and start a workout routine, you retain more fluid, and your weight might not exactly reflect calories burned. Tracking your progress by how your clothes fit and testing your body fat percentage is a better measure for overall fitness. Chapter 3 covers tracking your progress with body fat percentage.

Tracking calories burned

To help take the guesswork out of how many calories you burn through exercise, a host of products on the market do it for you, using sensors. Advanced ones also measure heart rate. After entering basic information about your height, weight, and age, a device like my favorite, FitBit, attaches to your clothing and tracks your daily steps taken, distance, and caloric expenditure. When worn at night, it also tracks your sleeping efficiency. All this info is then uploaded to your computer for viewing, adding custom activity, and tracking your progress over time. Being able to measure this is motivation in itself — you may find yourself wanting to take those extra steps to walk to the grocery store just to see the number increase on the device (I know I have!). If you aren't able to do regular exercise, just monitor your steps per day with a device like this or a standard pedometer; aim for 10,000 steps per day for a solid amount of daily activity.

Your best friend, the afterburn

Although the fat-burning zone during exercise is somewhat of a misnomer, the idea of an afterburn is very real. When you're exercising, your body is working hard to do a variety of tasks at once, and when you stop, your body then goes through a process to normalize itself.

This normalization is also known as *excess post-exercise oxygen consumption*, or EPOC. The longer and more intense the activity, the more oxygen your body takes up to replenish your cells. This translates into more calories burned throughout the day and a boosted metabolic rate.

A study published in *Medicine and Science in Sports and Exercise* found that 45 minutes of vigorous cycling exercise increased metabolic rate for up to 14 hours post workout. The young men in the study burned about 190 calories more during the rest of the day — not including calories burned during exercise. The effect is also seen with short bouts of resistance exercise; one study found that this can keep the afterburn going for up to 48 hours later!

The amount of calories you can actually burn will vary significantly depending on length of exercise, your body composition, age, and even outdoor temperature. But the highest post-exercise calorie burn occurs when your heart rate is within the zone of 70–85 percent of your max. This means the fat-burning zone of lower intensity exercise I mentioned earlier doesn't necessarily burn more fat in the long haul.

If you're not measuring your heart rate, vigorous-intensity activity with a max after burn means the following:

- ✔ At minimum, it's ten minutes long.

- ✔ You're short of breath and can only speak a few words at a time — also known as the *talk test* (with moderately intense exercise, you're able to talk but not sing).

- ✔ You're probably sweating.

- ✔ You're jogging, running, swimming laps, cycling more than 10 miles per hour, hiking uphill, speed walking, or playing sports with lots of running like soccer, singles tennis, or basketball.

The longer and more frequently you do these activities, the better. But you also need to be aware of another kind of burn: burning out. It may not be realistic for you to do an hour per day, and that's okay. The rest of this chapter walks you through putting a plan in place, listening to your body, and mixing up your workouts in ways that will work for you.

If you know you can't do high- or even moderate-intensity exercise due to an injury or weakness, you can still reap the benefits of additional calories burned by doing low-intensity exercise like walking or leisurely swimming. Just tack on more time to your workout to maximize how much you can burn.

Finding Your Inner Athlete

Two of the hardest things about making lifestyle changes with diet and exercise are being in the right mindset and getting started. Be proud of yourself! You've picked up this book, and somewhere, maybe deep down, that means you're motivated. You *can* reach your goals, whatever they are, wherever you're at.

Personally, I've come a long way with regard to fitness. As any of my childhood friends will tell you, I was the most uncoordinated, slowest, klutz there was. I was picked last for teams and was usually the reason we lost the game. It wasn't until college that I truly found my inner athlete. As a way to burn stress (not calories) from a heavy science-based nutrition workload, I begin jogging outdoors.

It started as a mile here and there, but then I carved out a regular time for running within a hectic schedule. It was an epiphany for me when I started not only being less stressed, but sleeping better and feeling loads more energy. I slowly increased mileage and, after about a year, was running far enough that a marathon was well within reach.

I'm not saying you have to start running marathons — I only ran one and currently run only a few miles per week. What I'm talking about is building the time in for activity just as you would for a meal or for watching your favorite television show. You don't eat the same exact food at every meal and you don't watch the same episode over and over. What makes it enjoyable is that they are different experiences that affect you in different ways. Why not approach activity with the same mindset?

Being consistent

In many ways, the *fact* that you engage in activity is even more important than exactly *what* you're doing for activity. The next section contains many exercises you can do to maximize your calorie burn. You don't have to do every single one every day, but putting together a workout plan that will be realistic for you to do on a regular basis is your number one priority right now.

The definition of *consistent activity* will likely vary throughout your life. Maybe you can make time for an hour of planned exercise every day, or three times per week, or once per week. If you can't do it at all, be consistent with parking your car farther from your destination so you walk a bit more, do regular house cleaning, or take the stairs instead of the elevator — they all count as calories burned and can add up.

Increase your chances for consistency for exercise with these steps:

✔ **Be a goal setter (both short term and long term):** This will help keep your eyes on the prize and stay motivated. An example of a long-term goal is to reduce your body fat percentage. A short-term goal for a novice can be to walk or jog one mile every other day. Once you complete the task, mark it off on your calendar with a big checkmark for the visual motivation. As you complete each short-term goal, picture how it will affect your long-term goal.

✔ **Be a realist:** You're probably not going to do every single exercise in this chapter every day right off the bat. Create a calendar and insert chunks of time with corresponding activities you can do at that time. If you don't follow through some days, you're not undoing all of your positive efforts — just get right back to it as soon as you can. But the more you stick to it, the easier it will become. Be patient and kind with yourself.

✔ **Be a troubleshooter:** Identify what barriers are in place for your exercise plan right away and adjust accordingly. If you find you're more likely to overeat on days you exercise, then plan the timing or composition of your meals in anticipation of that. Or if you find that a routine you've put into place is just not working for you, you feel too tired or are struggling with injury, or you're just bored of staring at the screen on the elliptical machine, it's time to make a change so it's more stimulating, realistic, and sustainable for you.

Keeping your body guessing to avoid the plateau

When I first started running, I saw results mentally and physically. But over time, because I was doing more or less the same activity day in and day out, without changing it up, I came to a plateau. The results I was seeing diminished, and I found it more and more difficult to push myself harder.

Although being consistent with doing activity is important, so that it becomes habitual for you to make the time for it, you don't want your body to get into the habit of doing the same activity over and over. Your body and muscles become adjusted to all they know they have to handle.

Think about it this way: If you have a job that involves repetitive tasks, and you know exactly what you're going to do every day, you may not be stimulated anymore. You basically work on autopilot. That's how your muscles may handle a repetitive task. They get bored, and your growth comes to a halt.

Surprise your muscles to keep them guessing about the work they'll perform that day. That way, they'll work harder, more efficiently, and your strength and endurance will definitely benefit. When you keep it interesting, you'll also feel stimulated in different ways, see results, and therefore be more likely to keep it up:

- ✔ **Exercise surprise:** If you've done the same cardio for years at a time, you need to mix it up (see the next section for a variety of exercises to try out). Be creative with how you move your body and work out different muscle groups than usual. If you're a devout runner, try yoga. If all you do is lift weights, try an energizing spin class.

- ✔ **Intensity surprise:** When weight-lifting, increase the number of reps or sets that you do so your muscles recognize it's time to increase their strength to keep up. If you run on the treadmill, try sprinting at intervals or increasing the elevation during commercials. When listening to music, amp up intensity during each chorus of a song (I do this when running outdoors).

- ✔ **Rest surprise:** If you've hit a hard stop with results, you've overworked a muscle group or are bored with your routine and need a break — take it! Then when you start exercising again or go back to flexing a specific muscle group, it'll be shocked back into action.

Don't overdo it!

Just as your mind needs a break after a hectic day at work, your muscles need rest when intensely exercising to repair and maximize strength. What's *intense* for you depends on how much you've trained in the past.

Don't try to keep up with others' routines. Listen to your body or else you'll be at increased risk for injury and illness. The benefits that exercise can offer can be undone with overtraining. Look for these signs that you may be working too hard and need to rest up:

- ✔ You have consistent aches and pains from overusing certain muscles or joints.

- ✔ Your endurance is lower than usual, and you find you're getting more fatigued more quickly during workouts. If you don't give your muscles time to recover, they'll feel heavier and heavier.

- ✔ You're getting sick frequently. Overtraining can drain your resources physically to fight off infections.

- ✔ You're unable to concentrate, easily irritable, or experience mood swings. Overtraining can drain your resources mentally and alter your hormones, just like not getting enough sleep.

- ✔ You have a chronically elevated heart rate — a surefire sign of working too hard. Also, it'll take your heart rate longer to normalize post exercise.

- ✔ For the ladies: You aren't getting your period. Too much exercise without fueling your body properly with nutrition can result in loss of menstruation.

Getting caught up in being enthusiastic about exercise is easy, especially if you're a newbie or have found exercises you love to do. But remember to listen to what your body is telling you so that you don't burn out quickly, injure yourself, or adversely affect your health.

Mixing It Up

Any fitness professional will tell you that one of the most important aspects of getting in shape is variety. That's not only because muscles begin to adapt to the same activity over time or because you shouldn't overtrain a specific region of your body, but because you'll get *bored* doing the same routine over and over. That's why a personal trainer has you do different activities and pushes you to do extra reps (even if you hate them in the process) — so that you reap all the benefits exercise can offer you and stay motivated to continue.

This section reviews the kinds of workouts you can do to maximize your metabolism's full potential. I break them down into different categories: cardio, weights, resistance, and alternative exercise.

If you've never exercised, have a chronic health condition, are a smoker, are older than 45 (man) or 55 (woman), or are overweight, you should see your doctor before engaging in any vigorous training or exercise.

Cardio

When you're just first starting out with a workout routine, cardiovascular exercise may be your way to go. We're talking about activity that gets your heart rate up and increases blood flow — not taking leisurely walks around the block. Aim to build up to being able to add these cardio levels into your routine.

✔ Moderate-intensity cardio: 30 minutes, 5 days per week

- Brisk walking

- Bike riding on level ground

- Water aerobics

✔ High-intensity cardio: 15–20 minutes, 5 days per week

- Jogging or running

- Cycling with hills

- Playing sports with running

- Swimming laps

- Interval training

If breaking up the workouts into a few 10-minute sessions is more realistic for you, go for it! A study published in the *Journal of Strength and Conditioning Research* found that breaking up workouts was even more effective for weight control and improvement of health markers in middle-aged men and women, mostly because these shorter sessions were more likely to be sustainable for the subjects in the study.

Whatever will keep you going is the best way to go.

For years, athletes have been on the interval training bandwagon to optimize their endurance and increase strength. High-intensity interval training (HIIT) combines intense bursts of activity like sprinting or climbing hills with periods of recovery — either rest or lower-intensity activities. If you think about it, it's perfect conditioning for sports such as basketball, which combines quick movement for running down the court and breaks when setting up for a shot, sitting on the bench, timeouts, and so on.

You don't have to be an athlete to reap the benefits of HIIT. HIIT is touted as the best way to burn the most calories and increase fat oxidation within one workout. Usually, since these types of workouts are harder, they last for shorter sessions — about 20 minutes — than typical cardio workouts. However, you get a lot of bang for your buck with HIIT:

✔ You burn more calories per session than you would with lower-intensity activity.

✔ You improve your heart's ability to carry oxygen to your muscles, increasing cardiovascular ability.

✔ You maximize your endurance with less muscle fatigue over time.

Don't forget to warm up before intense exercise. A warmup increases blood flow, reduces risk for injury, and prepares you both mentally and physically for the energy you're about to expend. You can warm up with 5–10 minutes of a lighter activity such as a brisk walk or a jog, or doing some flexibility work. Cooling down post exercise with the same type of movements for the same amount of time can help prevent muscle stiffness and improve recovery.

If you're a beginner, HIIT is not the first type of activity you want to try to do, but it can be something you build up to. Once you have several weeks of activity under your belt or once getting regular exercise is already a habit for you, then you can consider focusing on the intensity and length of your workouts.

Here's an example of a 20-minute HIIT cardio routine that can be adapted to any fitness level:

1. Warm up. Lightly jog for 5 minutes.

2. Run for 1 minute at a moderate or high intensity.

3. Jog for 1 minute at low intensity.

4. Repeat steps 2 and 3 for 5 or 6 times.

5. Cool down. Lightly jog for 3–5 minutes.

Don't forget that if you sprint to catch a bus, that's like doing a mini interval workout in your daily life! Intervals can also include light weight-lifting or resistance work during rest or recovery periods instead of doing the cardio at a lower rate. So, if you're doing housework with periods of heavy gardening, vacuuming, or raking, that all counts towards an increased calorie burn. Or you can incorporate exercises from the next section into a cardio workout routine to mix it up.

Weight-lifting and resistance

Although most newbies to exercise start with cardio or aerobic workouts, you don't have to be a muscle man to incorporate weights and resistance into your regular activity or routine. Weights and resistance work help build and define muscle and improve bone density, posture, and flexibility. In addition to building physical strength, you're also working your brain muscle. Being stronger can give you more confidence, and research also shows it can help prevent age-related decline in cognitive function. Finally, using weights and your body for resistance complements the cardio you do to improve your muscles' ability to use oxygen, stabilize blood glucose, and maximize your metabolic rate.

Without incorporating muscle training, you can lose about 5 pounds of muscle per decade after 30 years of age! This can translate to you burning about 30 calories less per day every year. That might not sound like a lot, but it can add up to about 10 pounds gained per decade if you're not changing your diet. It's never too late to reverse the trend by incorporating full-body muscular work about 2 days per week at about 20–30 minutes each session.

Whether you want moves that tackle multiple muscles or ones that isolate them, I've got you covered on proper form with some of my favorites. However, I give preferential treatment to moves that don't require any equipment so that they can be done anytime, anywhere.

In general, you can do three *sets* (10–12 repetitions) of an exercise with 1 minute of rest between each set. When it comes to dumbbells, choose a weight that will cause you to tire after one set of the exercise. For women, 3–5 pounds in each hand is a great start; for men, 8–10 pounds in each hand. As you get stronger, you'll need to increase the weight incrementally.

Negative training for positive rewards

Negative training doesn't mean having a negative attitude when you're lifting weights. It means not sloughing off the importance of the second half of the motion when using weights. For example, if you're doing a bicep curl with weights, you may lift up and then release your hands back down to your sides quickly. Negative training says to stay in control of the movement the entire time — take the weights up in 3 to 5 counts, and down in 3 to 5 counts. Your muscle can actually handle more weight on the way down (lengthening) then on the way up (contracting), so exploiting negative training is like adding an extra set for those muscles.

You can even use a spotter to help you lift the weights up for you so that you can only practice the negative side and use more resistance. Or use both limbs on the positive, and one at a time when lengthening back. Because negative exercise causes more tension and muscle tearing, more protein synthesis is required to rebuild, resulting in higher calorie burn and increased strength. Remember though, that you have to replenish those muscle stores post-workout. Choosing a snack or meal of lean protein and carbohydrate within 30 minutes of weight sessions will do the trick!

Full Body Exercises

When you're short on time, you can make the most of the weight or resistance work that you do using exercises that work multiple muscles of your body.

Dumbbell front squat

These work your full body but can also be done without weights if you don't have them for an anytime workout on-the-go for your legs. **Targets:** full body, back, butt/hips, thighs. See Figure 11-1.

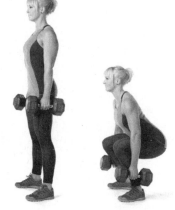

Figure 11-1: Dumbbell front squat.

Photographs by Bob McNamara

1. **Starting position:** Stand up tall with your feet slightly wider than hip-width apart. Roll your shoulders up to your ears and pull them back. Hold a dumbbell in each hand with your palms facing towards you.

2. **Squat:** Hinge at your hips, lower them back and down and bend your knees as if you're sitting in a chair. Take a look down and make sure your knee doesn't travel past your big toe (you should see your big toe when you look down). Your thighs should be parallel to the floor and your legs at a 90 degree angle. Keep your back flat.

3. **Lift up:** Keeping your abdominals engaged, lift up to starting position. Push through your heels and keep them flat on the floor.

Modification (easier): If these are too difficult or you need more security, use a chair as a guide or to sit in briefly at the bottom of the squat.

Modification (more difficult): As shown in Figure 11-2, you can also curl the dumbbells up to your shoulders and shift more weight into your heels to increase the intensity of the exercise and be able to squat more deeply.

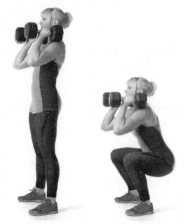

Figure 11-2:
Dumbbell
front squat
modified.

Photographs by Bob McNamara

Always keep your abdominals engaged during exercise to protect your spine.

Dumbbell lunge

You can either do these standing in one place or, for a bit of variety and to give yourself an end marker, while moving across a room. **Targets:** full body, abs, butt/hips, thighs. See Figure 11-3.

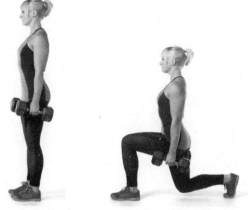

Figure 11-3:
Dumbbell
lunge.

Photographs by Bob McNamara

1. **Starting position:** Stand up tall with your feet about hip-width apart. Roll your shoulders up to your ears and down your back while engaging your abs (like always!).

2. **Lunge forward:** Keep your left foot planted firmly into the ground and lift your right foot off the floor. Take a big step forward with your right foot, heel first, and lower yourself down until your thigh is parallel with the floor. Push back with your left foot through your heel and keep your hips squared forward. Keep your chest up and look straight ahead.

3. **Lift up:** Push off through the heel of your right foot and lift back up to starting position. Keep working on one side or alternate between the two until you've completed 10 reps on each side.

I provide repetition guidelines in these exercises, but these are just guidelines — numbers you should be aiming for, not necessarily the amount of reps you will be doing from the get-go. In this example, you can start with 2 on each side and build up from there.

For more variety, with either a dumbbell in each hand or with a medicine ball held between your palms at the center of your chest, press the weight overhead as you come down into your lunge forward. Or for just a lower body workout, ditch the weight.

Spider walk

With no equipment necessary and only a little bit of floor space, the spider walk uses your own body's resistance to work your entire body. It may seem awkward at first, but once you get it down, you have an exercise you can do anytime, anywhere! **Targets:** arms (triceps), butt, abs, legs. See Figure 11-4.

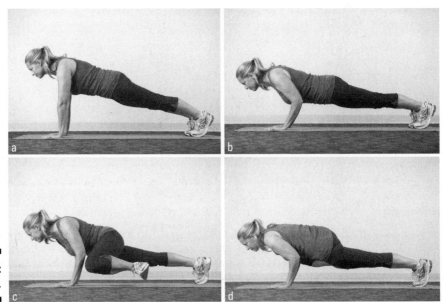

Figure 11-4: Spider walk.

Photographs by Matt Bowen

1. **Starting position:** Lie on your stomach with your hands below your shoulders. Point your fingers forward and keep your elbows close to the side of your body. Look straight ahead, keep your shoulders pulled back and your abdominals engaged.

2. **Crawl:** Bend and drive your right knee forward out to the right side so that it's level with your right hip or touches your right elbow. Place your foot on the floor. Lift up your left hand and move it forward the same distance your right foot traveled. From here, move the opposing limbs in the same fashion (left leg, right arm). Repeat 10 times on each side.

Modification: To increase the intensity, increase the number of reps or increase the speed at which you move.

Medicine ball squats

Using a medicine ball and a wall, you can get in a full body workout that's fun and boosts your heart rate. **Targets:** glutes, hips, thighs, arms, and core. See Figure 11-5.

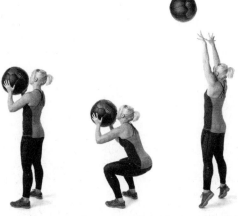

Figure 11-5: Medicine ball squats.

Photographs by Bob McNamara

1. **Starting position:** Start standing about 2 feet away from a wall, feet shoulder-width apart. Hold a medicine ball between the palms of your hands, starting out with a weight of 5 or 10 pounds.

2. **Squat and jump:** Lower your legs into a squat position, keeping the ball at chin level. Quickly jump up, onto your toes, and toss the ball against the wall about 2 feet above the height of your head. Your body should be fully extended at the top with your arms pointing toward the ball target.

3. **Catch and repeat:** As the ball bounces off the wall, catch it close to your chin, land softly back on your heels, and transition right into the next repetition of squatting and jumping. The movement should be fluid and controlled. Aim for 10–12 reps, rest for a minute, and repeat 2 or 3 times.

 Don't forget to breathe! Always exhale on the exertion, as you're jumping, sitting, or moving upward during any exercise. If you ever feel faint or short of breath, stop and rest until you can catch it again.

Upper Body and Core

If you pair upper-body strength exercises with cardio that involves resistance work, such as going uphill, you can get a full-body workout. Breaking exercises down by area of the body can help you mix it up without overtraining one muscle set. *Core*, or abdominal, exercise is integral to almost every movement because it helps with so much: balance, coordination, and flexibility. It also improves your performance with cardio workouts. Although your abs may recover more quickly than other muscles, remember that they still need rest too.

Your triceps muscles are located on the back of your arm from elbow to shoulder. Did you know that the triceps account for over half of the total muscle in your arm? Now that you do, what are you gonna do about it? These exercises can help you tone and build that large muscle.

Triceps kickback

1. **Starting position:** Stand up in split-stance position, with your right leg forward, holding a dumbbell in your left hand. Place your right hand on your right thigh and slowly lean forward to 45 degrees while keeping your head in line with your spine. Keeping your left arm close to your body, bend your left elbow so that your forearm is vertical to the floor. Keep your abs engaged.

2. **Kickback:** Extend and straighten your elbow while keeping your upper arm close to your torso. Slowly bend to bring back to starting and repeat.

 Modification: For more advanced kickbacks, keep your feet together, use a weight in each hand, and lean over so that your torso is parallel to the floor. Or for more support, use a weight bench as shown in Figure 11-6 and place your opposite knee on the bench.

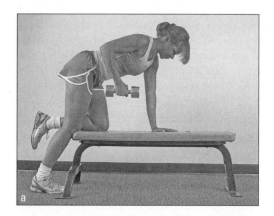

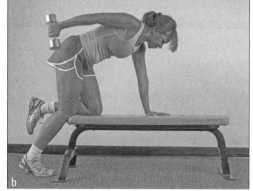

Figure 11-6:
Triceps
kickback

Photographs by Matt Bowen

Triceps dip

I love these because you don't need any weights to do them. You can dip
from a chair, a couch, or even the floor.

1. **Starting position:** Sit on a chair with your hands gripping the edge of the
   seat, fingers pointed in front of you. Extend your legs out in front of you
   with your heels on the ground.

2. **Dip:** Pull your butt off the edge of the front of the chair. Bend at the elbow
   to lower your body straight down until your elbows are at a 90 degree angle.
   Keep your arms in close to your body and your buttocks close to the chair.

3. **Push up:** Push back up and repeat 10–12 times. Rest on the chair as needed.

 To dip off the ground, come to a seated position with your legs extended in
front of you. Place your hands on the floor behind you, fingertips pointed
facing forward. Lift your buttocks up off the ground and walk your feet out to a
comfortable distance. Dip down by bending your elbows only. For a more
advanced move, lift one leg up at a time.

Push-up progression

You can do push-ups anywhere. The push-up is one of the best exercises for arm strength while working your entire body. Don't be intimidated — you can start on your knees and then build up to regular pushups on the balls of your feet. **Targets:** arms, butt/hips, chest, shoulder, core, full body. See Figure 11-7.

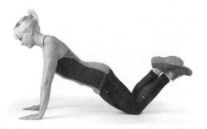

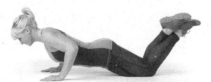

Figure 11-7: Modified push-up.

Photographs by Bob McNamara

1. **Starting position:** Go down on your hands and knees and place your hands on the floor directly beneath your shoulders, fingers facing forward. Adjust your knees so that your torso is in a straight line with your head, with no bend in your hips.

2. **Down and up:** Keeping your elbows close to your body, slowly bend them to lower your body to the floor (just touching or hovering above) without allowing your hips to sag. Imagine you have a cup of water on your lower back. Push back up, maintaining that same rigidity.

Plank: To do a regular push-up, start in plank position (Figure 11-8). Get on your hands and knees with your hands directly under your shoulders, fingers facing forward. Extend one leg and then the other behind you so that your feet are together, toes tucked, heels reaching way back. Your head and spine should be aligned. Engage your core throughout the exercise to protect your lower back. See Figure 11-9.

Holding in plank pose can help define your abdominal muscles and prevent back injury. For an easier pose, come down to your forearms. For a more difficult plank pose, lift one leg up at a time and hold for 10 seconds before switching legs.

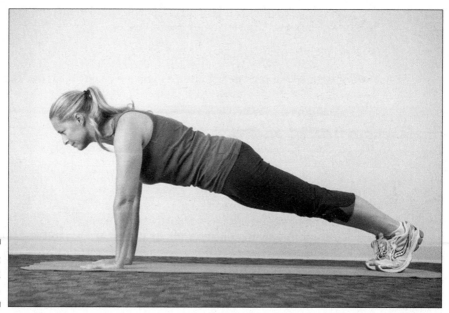

Figure 11-8:
Plank
position.

Photograph by Matt Bowen

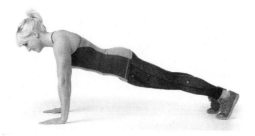

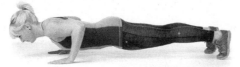

Figure 11-9:
Regular
push-up.

Photographs by Bob McNamara

When doing a regular push-up, you can either bend your elbows out to the
sides which will work more of your chest and back muscles or keep your
elbows close to your body to work the triceps.

If you've mastered the standard push-up, you can add instability so that you're working even more of your core muscles:

- Place a medicine ball under one hand on the floor.
- Alternate keeping one leg lifted as you lower down to the floor.

Spinning planks

Building on what you learned with the previous description of planks, you can try this more advanced full-body exercise that uses your own body weight for resistance. See Figure 11-10.

1. **Starting position:** Start in a plank position as in Figure 11-8. Shift your weight to the right side and rotate your left arm up to the ceiling while balancing on your right foot. For a more advanced pose, lift your left leg slightly. Hold for 5–10 seconds (one-one-thousand, two-one-thousand, and so on).

2. **Flip:** Continue to rotate your left arm back to the floor so that your stomach is facing the ceiling. Push your hips up and tighten your core so that your hips don't sag. This is a reverse plank.

3. **Reverse:** Now, keep your left arm on the ground and begin to rotate your right arm up so you're in a side plank on the opposite side. Hold for the same amount of time you did on the right side. Return to standard plank position. Lower your knees if you need to rest. Otherwise complete 5 full rotations.

Dumbbell press

This is my go-to all-around arm and back strength exercise. If you don't have weights you can add resistance by taking an old t-shirt, twisting it up until it's a straight line, and holding each end with one hand, close enough so there's tension. My friend and fitness professional, Kim Fleming, taught me that tip. See Figure 11-11.

1. **Starting position:** Lie on your back with your knees bent so that your feet are flat on the ground. Hold one weight in each hand and bring them in front of your chest. Your upper arms should be parallel to the floor (either resting on the floor or hovering slightly above) and your lower arms vertical, palms facing away.

2. **Press:** Press the dumbbells upward until your arms are fully extended and parallel to each other. You can rotate your palms to face each other at the top. Slowly lower dumbbells back to starting position and repeat.

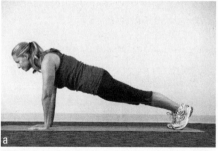
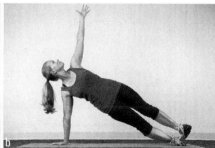
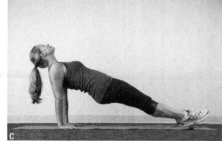

Photographs by Matt Bowen

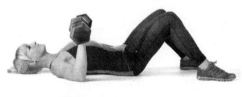
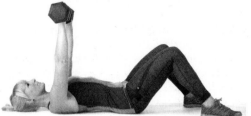

Photographs by Bob McNamara

Supine bicycle crunches

These are the most fun abdominal exercises in my opinion, and yes, I'm being serious. These are also effective for working your abdominal muscles, including your *obliques*, which are the sides of your core. See Figure 11-12.

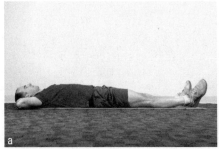
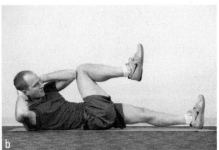

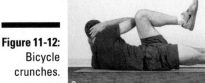
Figure 11-12:
Bicycle
crunches.

Photographs by Matt Bowen

1. **Starting position:** Lie flat on the floor with your lower back pushing into the floor and hands behind your head. Bend your knees and lift your legs up to a 90 degree angle so your thighs are perpendicular to the floor.

2. **Bicycle and twist:** Simultaneously bring your right knee into your right armpit and extend your left leg out straight at a 45 degree angle to the floor. Rotate your torso to bring your left elbow towards your right knee. Hold this position for a moment, then alternate.

Don't pull forward on your neck. Instead, make sure to keep your elbows back and your hands just lightly supporting the back of your head. To minimize risk of injury, focus on lifting and twisting your core to do the work. Hold in your abdominals to protect your spine.

Trying Exercise Classes

Taking exercise classes is great. You can discover new movements that speak to you, learn proper technique from an instructor, and stay engaged with a variety of workouts. I also strongly encourage you to take classes or personal training sessions for weights and other aerobic exercises. I think of Pilates and yoga together because I believe you should learn them from a real live teacher, plus being in a class can help you connect with other like-minded people. Yoga may sound New Agey to you, but it's been around for centuries and is definitely not a fad.

Yoga

Yoga is not only for spiritual peace of mind — it can be super hard. There are many different kinds of yoga, from Bikram (hot yoga) to Hatha (slow poses, good for beginners) to Vinyasa (more fast-paced, flowing movements). They all have benefits for mind and body, relaxation, flexibility, and improving your metabolic rate.

Sun Salutation

The Sun Salutation is a series of poses which helps get your body warmed up and is a good one to do first thing in the morning, before any workout — or any time you need a full body stretch. See Figure 11-13.

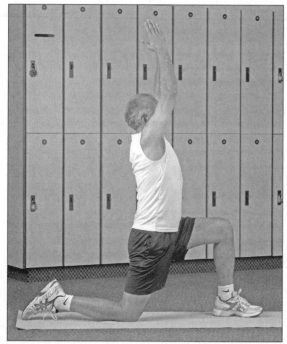

Figure 11-13:
Basic Sun
Salutation.

Photograph by Matt Bowen

1. **Starting position:** Kneel on the floor and bring your left foot forward so it's flat and bent at a 90 degree angle, with your thigh parallel to the floor.

2. **Lift:** Touch your palms together and lift your arms straight up. Engage your abdominals and keep your shoulders down and back.

3. **Stretch:** Look to the ceiling as you stretch upward with your upper body and shift your weight to your front thigh. Repeat with your right leg forward.

Triangle Pose

This pose is one of my favorites in yoga class. It works to stretch out your abdomen and spine. See Figure 11-14.

Figure 11-14:
Triangle
Pose.

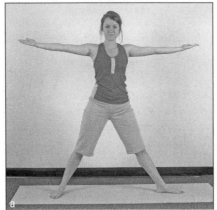 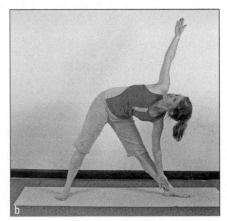

Photographs by Matt Bowen

1. **Starting position:** Stand with your feet much wider than your shoulders and place both arms out to your sides, palms facing up, parallel to the floor.

2. **Bend and stretch:** Keeping your legs straight and hips facing forward, bend at your waist to your right side. Slide your arm down your right leg and hold your leg and ankle. Take five deep breaths. Lift up and repeat on opposite side.

Downward Facing Dog

This is a *restorative pose*, meaning during a yoga session, you come back to it frequently to stretch your entire body. See Figure 11-15.

1. **Starting position:** Start on your hands and knees. Your knees should be directly under your hips and your hands slightly in front of your shoulders.

2. **Lift:** Slowly lift your knees away from the floor and lengthen your tailbone up until your body forms an upside-down V shape.

3. **Stretch:** Straighten your knees and either keep your heels slightly lifted or place on the ground depending on your flexibility. Roll your upper arms and upper thighs inward slightly. Firm your shoulder blades together and hold the position for five counts of deep breaths. Either return to start or move onto the next pose in your yoga sequence.

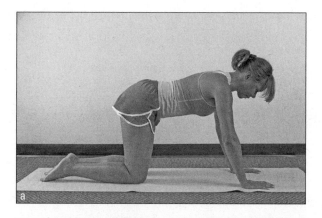

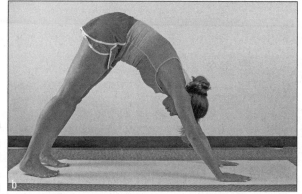

Figure 11-15:
Downward
Facing Dog.

Photographs by Matt Bowen

Bikram yoga, performed in a room heated to 100 degrees or more, is not for the faint of heart. Before trying it, check with your doctor if you have a history of heart or respiratory disease, diabetes, or if you're pregnant. You need to drink water before, during, and after, and you need to wear lighter clothing. If you feel faint, dizzy, or weak, stop immediately!

Pilates

Pilates, like yoga, works all muscles in your body to improve your strength and ability with any exercise. Unlike traditional yoga, equipment is commonly used in Pilates, such as the Reformer, which helps optimize the moves and your posture, spine flexibility, and core strength. However, there are also mat classes, which can benefit you in more ways than one.

Pilates 100 is a classic exercise that works your core better than crunches. See Figure 11-16.

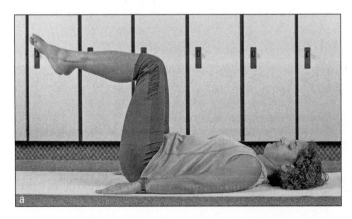

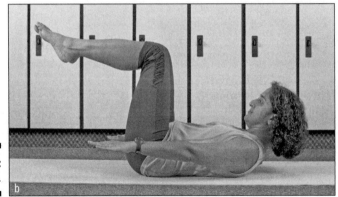

Figure 11-16:
Pilates 100.

1. **Starting position:** Lie on your back and bring your knees to a 90 degree angle to your upper thighs. Extend your arms along your sides, palms facing down. Pull your belly in and inhale.

2. **Round up and pump:** Exhale and slowly begin to round up to bring your chin towards your chest. Lift your arms about three inches off the floor, keeping them straight and rigid. Pump them up and down repeatedly. Only let your arms rise to slightly above your body. Inhale for a count of five and exhale for five until you reach 100 pumps total. Hug your knees into your chest to stretch.

Modification: For a more advanced Pilates 100, extend your legs out straight to 45 degrees or an even lower, more challenging angle.

The martial arts are another spiritual form of exercise for mind and body. Tai chi and Qi gong focus on the _Qi_ in Chinese culture, which means _energy flow_ or _life source_. Instead of working on complex movements, the focus is on breathing and concentration. For a low-impact workout that can help improve relaxation, balance, agility, and strength, try out one of these classes!

Sample Slimming Workouts

Whether you have ten minutes or are lucky enough to have one or even two hours per day to exercise, you want to make the most of your time. The strength routines in this section are designed to help you boost your caloric burn while mixing up the muscle groups being worked. You can swap out exercises from the same section to create even more routines to stay entertained and fired up about working out. You can do the ones in Table 11-2 anytime, anywhere.

Table 11-2	Ten-Minute Power Blast	
Time	**Activity**	**Notes**
2 minutes	Warm-up	Jog in place, brisk walk, Sun Salutations
1 minute	Squats	With or without dumbbells
2 minutes	Jumps	Try jumping jacks or jump rope
1 minute	Triceps	Kickbacks with weights or dips without
2 minutes	Spinning planks	Get that heart rate up!
2 minutes	Bicycle crunches	Or any other abdominal exercise

Don't poo-poo the ten-minute workout. It's better to do any minutes than none. Every minute you burn more calories than you would at rest counts. Do ten minutes once, twice, or three times per day to get your heart rate up and work those muscles. However, if you have 30 minutes, try the next routine.

A recent study published in the _American Journal of Physiology_ found that exercising for 30 minutes per day may be even better than exercising for one hour. Participants who were previously sedentary and worked out 30 minutes per day — despite burning half the calories as they would have in 60 minutes — lost the same amount of body fat and weight.

The authors speculate, and I agree, this may be because people were more likely to stay engaged with a 30-minute workout and perhaps ate less to compensate for less activity. So, if you're the type of person who may eat more when working out a lot, start with the 30-minute routines in Table 11-3.

Table 11-3		30 Minutes to Burn
Time (min.)	*Activity*	*Notes*
1	Plank pose	On your forearms or full plank
3	Medicine Ball Squats	Or just plain squats
1	Push-ups	Any variation of your choosing
3	Dumbbell lunges	Alternating each side
1	Plank pose	Try lifting up each leg for 30 seconds
3	Jumping rope	If you don't have one, pretend!
1	Pilates 100s	Or bicycle crunches
3	Reverse dumbbell lunges	Instead of stepping forward, step back
1	Push-ups	Challenge yourself with leg lifts or one hand on a medicine ball
3	Jumping rope	Land lightly and twist your hips side to side
1	Triangle Pose	
3	Repeat any of these!	
1	Bicycle Crunches	Or Pilates 100
3	Repeat any of these!	
2	Cool down with yoga poses, walking, or any stretch you like	

If you have an hour to exercise, try doing a 30-minute strength routine paired with 30 minutes of moderate cardio like bicycling, jogging, brisk walking, or swimming. Or if you're cardio-ed out, pair with a mind-body exercise class like yoga. That way you get all the exercise benefits without the risk of overworking yourself physically or mentally.

Stretch it out! Post workout or even as a lower intensity form of movement, stretching out your muscles can improve your flexibility, prevent injury, and keep the blood flowing to all parts of your body. Stretching can also be super relaxing — just make sure that you follow these tips:

✔ Stretch each muscle used during the workout.

✔ Hold each stretch position for 15–30 seconds.

✔ Avoid bouncing within the stretch — it can cause your muscles to overstrain.

✔ Stretch out warm muscles — either after you've warmed up already or post workout.

For much more information on stretching poses and benefits, check out *Stretching for Dummies* by LaReine Chabut and Madeleine Lewis (Wiley, 2007).

Your Weekly Exercise Calendar

What you're able to fit into your weekly exercise calendar will vary based on your work and family schedule. Make your own realistic schedule and write it down so you're more likely to stick to it. Table 11-4 gives you a sample for how to spread out your workouts.

Table 11-4	Sample Week of Exercise	
Day	**Activity**	**Time (min.)**
Sunday	Rest your muscles	
Monday	Strength/aerobic	Upper body resistance/weights 30, jog 30
Tuesday	Cardio blast	Interval cardio 30
Wednesday	Lower body strength	Swim 30
Thursday	Brisk walking	60
Friday	Full body strength	10 per routine (2)
Saturday	Flexibility: yoga, pilates, stretching	60

Fueling Up Before and After Working Out

Fueling up properly for the exercise you're doing is a big deal — before, to give you energy to keep going, and after, to repair your muscles and improve your endurance for next time (see Table 11-5). You should always eat something before you exercise intensely (intervals, for example). Working out on an empty stomach will *not* increase fat burned. Follow these guidelines for fueling the best you can before and after you get your move on:

✔ Eat within 30 minutes to 2 hours before exercising. Either have a small snack (100–200 calories) within 30 minutes or closer to 300 calories within 1–2 hours before exercising.

✔ Eat something between 30–60 minutes after you're finished. How much you should eat after depends on your calorie allotment for the day and how many hours until your next meal.

✔ Even first thing in the morning, have a banana or a glass of skim milk before workout.

✔ Make sure to include a source of protein before a workout, such as low-fat dairy, nuts, or lean meats with a meal — especially if you're working out for a long period of time or doing any type of weight/resistance work.

✔ Avoid big meals with high fat or high protein right before you work out because your stomach needs more time to digest and you might feel cramping, nausea, and/or sluggish during the act.

✔ After a workout, choose carbohydrate and protein in a 4:1 ratio — for example, 40 grams of carbohydrate and 10 grams of protein.

✔ Research shows having low-fat chocolate milk — a combination of carbohydrate and protein — after exercise may be one of the best sources to refuel muscles and improve glycogen stores for next time.

✔ Follow the metabolism-boosting guidelines of eating balanced meals/ snacks every 4–5 hours to keep your body fueled all day long for all the activity that you do.

Table 11-5	Best Snacks for Working Out	
Calorie Level	Pre Workout	Post Workout
100	Large banana or 1 cup skim milk	6 ounces low-fat Greek yogurt or 3 tablespoons hummus with 10 baby carrots
200	Apple with 1 ½ tablespoons peanut butter or 1 cup oatmeal with ½ cup low-fat milk	1 ½ cups chocolate soy milk or light string cheese with 1 ounce whole-wheat crackers
300	Energy bar (>3 grams fiber, >6 grams protein, <18 grams sugar) or 1 ounce almonds, 1 ⅕ cup dried fruit	3 ounces turkey, 2 slices whole-wheat bread or protein smoothie made with 2 cups of berries and 1 cup low-fat yogurt

Water can't be left out of the equation. Staying hydrated keeps you energized and ensures that you can exercise for longer. A surefire way to know whether you're drinking enough water while exercising is to weigh yourself before and after without clothes on. If your weight change is more than 2 percent of starting, then next time, plan to drink a cup of water at least 15 minutes before and every 15–20 minutes during your workout.

Post exercise, you need to drink 16 ounces of water for every pound lost during. Everyone's total daily water needs are different, but if you take your body weight in pounds and divide by 2 — that's the about the amount of fluid you need in ounces. So if you're 160 pounds, you need 80 ounces of fluid per day approximately (from liquids and water-dense foods). Keep drinking up!

Chapter 12

Spotlight on Hormone-Disrupting Conditions

. . . .

In This Chapter

▶ Understanding how certain conditions impact your metabolism

▶ Changing diet and lifestyle

. . . .

*H*ave you tried everything in the proverbial book to lose weight but feel that because you're going through menopause or have an underlying disease that the odds are stacked against you? It's true that certain conditions affect your metabolism, your hormonal balance, and your ability to lose weight. But by understanding what's actually going on in your body, you can fight back with specific changes.

I know it's frustrating if eating and exercising the same as your spouse or friend yields slower results because of your condition. But that's the point, you'll have to make different choices with the foods you eat to boost your metabolism. That doesn't mean going on crash diets or creating highly restrictive meal plans — those can be damaging to you even more than others and may well have the opposite effect from what you want.

This chapter is organized by condition and covers diabetes, hypothyroidism, polycystic ovarian syndrome, and menopause.

This information isn't meant to substitute for any advice or medication prescribed by your physician. Think of it as background on what's going on inside your body and your dietitian's prescription for the diet guidelines to follow with each.

The Diabetes Connection

If you have diabetes mellitus, you may already know what a huge impact diet and exercise have on your blood glucose levels, your need for medication, as well as how you feel. When it comes to your metabolism, if you compare yourself to someone without diabetes who is very similar to you in age, size, and gender, the major difference between you is how your body responds to the carbohydrates you eat. A disruption in the action of the hormone insulin is responsible for this. But by being conscious of what you eat, getting exercise, and having regular check-ins with a physician, you have the power to control your diabetes and reduce complications.

If you have diabetes and don't pay attention to high blood sugar levels or see a physician about it, there can be serious repercussions on all parts of your body, not just your metabolism:

- ✔ **Feet:** Nerve damage and decreased circulation can result in foot ulcers and potentially amputation.

- ✔ **Eyes:** Retinopathy or decreased vision, glaucoma, and cataracts.

- ✔ **Skin:** Damage to blood vessels, bacterial or fungal infections.

- ✔ **Stomach:** From nerve damage to the muscles of the intestine over time, you can develop gastroparesis, which causes slower emptying of food and decreased digestion.

- ✔ **Heart:** About two thirds of adults with diabetes also suffer from high blood pressure and heart disease and are more likely to have a heart attack or stroke.

- ✔ **Kidneys:** Decreased kidney function from damage to your nerves.

- ✔ **Brain:** High or low blood glucose can affect your stress levels, ability to concentrate, make you prone to fatigue, and cause irritability.

Tracking glucose

A day in the life of a carbohydrate is different depending on whether you have diabetes. But your body's first goal is always the same: to break down the carbohydrate you eat into glucose so that your body can start using it for energy.

A carb needs to be broken down into simple sugars such as glucose, fructose, and galactose, to be absorbed and used by your body:

- ✔ Disaccharides are two or more of these simple sugars joined together. Examples are lactose (glucose + galactose), found in milk; sucrose (glucose + fructose), like table sugar; and maltose (glucose + glucose), or malt sugar from barley.

- ✔ Oligosaccharides are strands of 3–10 of these simple sugars.

- ✔ Polysaccharides are 10 or more joined together to create glycogen, starches, and fiber.

Your body wants to work as fast as it can to break down larger carbohydrate molecules into smaller ones so that it can use them for energy. Carbohydrates can begin digestion even before you swallow. Once you eat a slice of toast or a baked potato, starches from those foods immediately start getting broken down in your mouth by the enzyme amylase in your saliva. The breakdown continues through your digestive tract until the food hits the small intestine, where glucose molecules are absorbed by the bloodstream.

The next step is where having diabetes makes a difference to the metabolism of carbohydrate. It's the step where insulin takes the stage. This hormone does the following:

- ✔ Helps glucose get absorbed by the cells of your body for energy

- ✔ Promotes glucose to be linked up with other molecules to create glycogen, which is how carbohydrate is stored in your muscles and liver (for later use for energy)

- ✔ Slows the breakdown of fat and promotes fat storage

- ✔ Stimulates the creation of proteins from amino acids, which helps promote muscle growth

But when you have diabetes, your body can't do all that on its own. The two types of Diabetes are as follows:

- ✔ **Type 1:** Your pancreas stops producing insulin completely. This often occurs in childhood, and you're dependent on insulin therapy.

- ✔ **Type 2:** You have decreased insulin sensitivity, meaning your cells don't respond to insulin as they should and don't take up glucose for energy. This occurs for many reasons. It's often tied to obesity, but on a basic level it can be due to altered shape of insulin, decreased number of insulin receptors on the cells, or impaired communication. Typically diet, exercise, and oral hypoglycemic agents to increase your cells' response to insulin are prescribed.

With Type 2 on a cellular level, without taking medication or changing your diet and exercise, the following take place:

- ✔ Glucose can't be cleared from the bloodstream, but your cells feel deprived because they aren't getting the fuel. That makes you more likely to crave sweet foods.

- ✔ Once your glycogen stores are full, insulin converts that excess glucose floating around into fat.

- ✔ You'll have higher levels of circulating insulin, so your body thinks, "Oh, there's plenty of energy around," which impairs fat loss, increases triglycerides and fat storage, and decreases your ability to build muscle mass — all setbacks for your metabolic rate.

Don't take this as meaning you should avoid carbohydrates completely. Getting the right kinds is key to losing weight and keeping your energy levels high while doing so. Getting too few carbohydrates, especially if you're on medication, can result in low blood glucose with not-so-pretty side effects like heart palpitations, anxiety, and hunger. When you're brain isn't getting the glucose it needs, you can feel confused, and you suffer from headaches or more seriously, seizures.

Insulin sensitivity and glucose levels are directly impacted by diet, exercise, and your stress. When you get stressed, your blood glucose levels are even more elevated.

Go consistent with carbohydrates

Probably the most effective way to keep your blood glucose levels under control with diet is to count the carbohydrates you're taking in at every meal. Once you understand the science, it just may seem like common sense. Monitoring your carbohydrates and spreading them more evenly throughout the day helps your body best use them for energy without becoming overloaded.

A consistent carbohydrate diet means to have the same amount of carbohydrate servings at every meal. Doing this doesn't just help those with diabetes — it can help anyone trying to lose weight to boost their metabolism and help keep cravings under control, because your blood glucose levels are tried into cravings.

A serving of carbohydrates is 12–15 grams. If you're reading the Nutrition Facts Label for how many total carbohydrates there are in a food package, you must multiply the total number of carbohydrates by the number of servings in the package to arrive at the total in the entire package (assuming you're eating that much). Or dole out the allotted serving you need for that meal or snack.

Divvying up how many servings you need per meal is dependent on how many calories you take in throughout the day. Let's say you're on an 1,800 calories per day diet:

- About half your calories, or 900 calories, should come from carbohydrate.
- Because a carbohydrate gram is 4 calories (900 ÷ 4) = 225, you need about 225 grams of carbohydrate per day.
- You want to have three meals and two snacks per day to keep your blood glucose levels as stable as possible.
- Subtract 60 from 225 grams. Typically snacks should contain 1–2 servings, or 15–30 grams of carbohydrate each.
- That leaves you with 165 grams to divide among three meals. In general, having about 45–60 grams per meal (3 to 4 servings) is ideal. But it doesn't have to be exact. The goal is to spread out your carbohydrate intake throughout the day fairly evenly.

Ups and downs of the glycemic index (GI)

Carbohydrates raise your blood glucose levels by different degrees, depending on the type. The GI index measures just how high certain foods will raise your blood glucose compared to a reference food such as a slice of white bread.

Foods with a high GI raise your blood glucose more than those with a medium or low GI. The glycemic index isn't listed on the food label, and it's not always what you'd think. Carbohydrate foods with high fiber and any amount of protein are typically on the low end of the scale (because they slow absorption of sugar into your bloodstream), whereas refined carbohydrates are on the high end. Yes, in general the glycemic index gives you a good idea of which foods are nutritious and best for your blood sugar levels. On the other hand, some factors affect the GI and make it not the most plausible tool:

✔ Ripeness of fruits and veggies: The more ripe, the higher the GI

✔ Cooking time: The longer beans are cooked, the lower their GI

✔ Preparation: A mashed potato has a lower GI than a baked potato

✔ Type of grain: Oats, for example, have a high GI, which you may not expect because it's a whole grain and nutritious, whereas maple syrup has a lower GI

✔ What else is on the plate: The GI of your meal depends on what else you're eating

The bottom line is that you can't go just by the value of one food on its own. Also the GI index gives you no indication of how much you're consuming, so at the root, you've always got to count your carbs no matter what. Because low-GI foods don't raise your blood glucose as much, they can be great options to help you tweak your intake to optimize control. Research shows that people who consume a lot of high-GI foods do tend to have higher levels of body fat. However, it's not always practical to figure that out, and you may have just as much luck with weight loss and blood glucose control choosing high-fiber foods.

Counting carbohydrates may seem like a daunting task at first, but by making changes to your diet, you can improve your insulin sensitivity within days, and over time, reduce your need for medication. If you have diabetes, it's definitely worth it to become a carbohydrate-counting master. It'll help you keep portions in check, which will be good for weight loss as long as you're choosing foods that are also high in fiber, contain lean protein, as well as heart-healthy fats.

Learn what a serving of your favorite food is by reading the food label, especially for foods like sweets and snacks. You can also refer to Chapter 5 for sample exchanges in each of the carbohydrate-containing food groups, like fruits, vegetables, starches, and milk/yogurts.

When checking out a food label, look at total carbohydrates. Just because a product contains sugar alcohols doesn't mean it's sugar-free. Some of those alcohols (it's estimated about half) are actually absorbed like sugar into your bloodstream. However, a product with more fiber will work to minimize any blood glucose spikes.

Table 12-1 may make it just a little bit easier to understand what a serving is and what a sample meal plan can look like on an 1,800 calorie diet. For more on servings and carbohydrate counting, check out the American Diabetes Association at www.diabetes.org.

Table 12-1	Sample Diabetes Meal Plan	
Meal Time	*Food*	*Nutrition Count*
Breakfast	1 cup oatmeal, 1 teaspoon cinnamon, 1 cup low-fat plain yogurt, ¾ cup berries	350 calories, 60 grams carbs
Snack	1 cup sliced red pepper, 5 tablespoons hummus, 1 small apple	220 calories, 35 grams carbs
Lunch	Tuna fish sandwich on two slices whole-wheat bread, 1 ½ cup lentil soup	500 calories, 60 grams carbs
Snack	24 almonds, 1 cup skim milk	240 calories, 20 grams carbs
Dinner	1 ½ cups tossed salad, ½ tablespoon olive oil mixed with vinegar, 3 ounces grilled chicken, 1 medium baked sweet potato, 1 slice angel food cake	500 calories, 45 grams carbs
		Total: 1,810 calories, 220 grams carbs

Add a tablespoon of vinegar and a dash of cinnamon to your day. Research shows that these two condiments have benefits for blood glucose control. Vinegar may inhibit the digestion of starch so that blood glucose is less likely to spike after eating a meal. In addition, one study found that a gram of cinnamon per day can, over time, result in a 24 percent decrease in blood glucose levels. Other studies dispute this. But can it hurt? Probably not. Just let your doctor know if you consume vinegar or cinnamon so you can track the effects.

You may find your blood sugar is more difficult to control at a specific time of day. In that case, be extra cautious about the foods and servings that you eat at that time to optimize control. Getting exercise can also help clear glucose from your bloodstream because your muscles use it up for energy and your cells decrease their insulin resistance.

Aim for about 30 minutes of exercise on most days. The Diabetes Prevention Program study found that people with pre-diabetes (higher than normal blood sugar levels but not yet qualified for diabetes) were able to delay developing Type 2 diabetes with 150 minutes of exercise per week and diet changes. It doesn't have to be a chore — learn how to incorporate exercise easily into your day in Chapter 11.

Metabolic syndrome: A cluster of conditions

Also known as Syndrome X, metabolic syndrome is defined as several conditions that can increase your risk for diabetes and heart disease. These include: insulin resistance, high blood pressure, elevated blood glucose and lipid levels, tendency to develop blood clots, and too much fat around the waist. More than 30 percent of Americans (and rising) are thought to have metabolic syndrome. It's associated with obesity, although the two are not mutually inclusive. The truth is, there's no clear-cut definition or cause of metabolic syndrome, but many experts associate it with insulin resistance and symptoms of pre-diabetes. What can you do?

✔ Try to lose or maintain your weight so you're within 20 percent of your ideal body weight.

✔ Add more high-fiber foods and consume a consistent carbohydrate diet.

✔ Beans, beans are good for your heart. Research shows that beans can help lower blood pressure in diabetics and reduce risk for developing heart disease.

✔ Moderate your sodium intake by limiting table salt or commercially prepared foods.

✔ Reduce saturated fat intake from full-fat dairy and animal products.

✔ Choose heart-healthy fat sources like oils, fatty fish, nuts, seeds, and avocado.

✔ Start incorporating regular aerobic activity, about 20 minutes, into your day.

✔ Visit your physician for regular check-ups to monitor your vital signs and blood glucose levels.

✔ Mull over magnesium with your doctor. Studies have found that taking magnesium supplements can lower your risk for developing diabetes. Or go the natural route with magnesium-rich foods such as whole grains, nuts, and leafy green vegetables.

Talking About Thyroid Disease

If your metabolism is the engine of your body, your thyroid is a key that turns the ignition. The thyroid gland, located in your neck just below the Adam's apple, is responsible for producing hormones that regulate metabolism and growth. If the thyroid isn't working the way it should, that usually means the hormones it produces are out of whack. In this section, I talk about what your thyroid hormones do, the side effects of thyroid disease, and specific diet tips that may affect your thyroid.

Homing in on thyroid hormones

More than 20 million Americans produce too much (hyperthyroid) or too little (hypothyroid) hormones. Unfortunately, it's estimated that half of those people suffering don't even know it! If you've been doing everything you can to lose weight, experience the side effects discussed in this section, and suspect there's something else going on, visit a physician before assuming there's something wrong with your thyroid.

The hormones in question when we talk about *hyper-* versus *hypo-*thyroid disease are triidothyronine (T3) and thyroxine (T4). To produce them, your thyroid requires the element iodine, which you need to get through your diet. These hormones are triggered to be released when your pituitary gland releases Thyroid Stimulating Hormone (TSH). At that point, T3 and T4 help oxygen get into cells, where they do the following:

- ✔ Increase basal metabolic rate and body heat production
- ✔ Influence the rate of muscle growth and development
- ✔ Impact protein, fat, and carbohydrate metabolism
- ✔ Regulate synthesis of protein from amino acids
- ✔ Increase fat oxidation
- ✔ Assist absorption of glucose into cells as well as create free glucose
- ✔ Promote increased blood flow and mental acuity

If you have hyperthyroid or produce too much thyroid hormones, side effects include weight loss, anxiety, fast heartbeat, insomnia, muscle weakness, and increased bowel movements. But most people diagnosed with a thyroid condition — about 80 percent — have *hypo*thyroid. In this condition, your thyroid isn't producing enough hormones, and therefore your cells aren't able to convert calories into the energy they need to function the best they can.

If you have hypothyroidism, it's possible you're also dealing with one of these risk factors or symptoms:

- ✔ You've had unexplained weight gain.
- ✔ You're a female. (Females are 5–8 times more likely to develop thyroid conditions, especially during big hormonal changes like during pregnancy and menopause).
- ✔ You have a family history of thyroid disease or *goiters* (enlargement of the thyroid gland caused by iodine deficiency).
- ✔ You have high blood cholesterol levels.
- ✔ You're always cold.
- ✔ You're often sluggish and feel fatigued and depressed.
- ✔ You've had changes in your menstrual cycle.
- ✔ You're dealing with constipation or digestive issues.
- ✔ You've noticed you have dry skin, brittle hair and nails, or a puffy face.
- ✔ Your muscles are achy or you have pain or stiffness in joints.

It's clear that your thyroid and the hormones it produces are inextricably con-nected to your metabolic rate as well as how you look and feel. Once you've been diagnosed, your doctor will prescribe medication to treat your thyroid condition, but naturally diet plays a role as well.

Making your diet thyroid-friendly

Because your thyroid condition affects your weight and all aspects of your metabolism, this entire book was written for you. Following the metabolism-boosting basics — including the foods you want to limit or choose and sample meal plans in Chapters 4–6, will greatly benefit you, too. Of course, sleeping well and regular activity bring together many pieces of the puzzle.

Ditch the 1,000-calorie crash diets. Restricting calories too much slows down your metabolism, and often your weight won't budge. Your body is in a type of survival mode where it starts storing fat instead of burning it, and you lose more of your lean muscle mass to compensate. It's possible that with a thyroid condi-tion, this effect is exacerbated. See Chapter 3 to find out how many calories you need to eat to lose weight and keep your metabolism furnace burning.

Although medication helps regulate your hormones, there are still aspects of your diet to be aware of. *Goitrogens* refers to any food that impacts how your thyroid works by blocking iodine uptake. Your thyroid needs iodine to create hormones, so, without it, hormone production diminishes too. It's important to note that most cases of hypothyroid in the United States are caused by autoimmune diseases like Hashimoto's thyroiditis, and not from a deficiency in iodine.

Go slow with soy

Soybeans contain an antioxidant called isoflavone. Isoflavones may compete with the thyroid in getting iodine to create your hormones. A review of studies published in *Thyroid* concluded that soy supplementation and excess con-sumption of soy (especially in people who are iodine deficient, see later in this section) can slow your thyroid function and also can reduce the effect of your medication.

✔ Avoid soy or isoflavone supplements, protein powders, and pills.

✔ Try to limit genetically modified (GMO) soybeans, which are found in a plethora of products from cereals to processed meats.

✔ Choose soy that's fermented or cooked — this may decrease the nega-tive effects. Cooked tofu or soybeans and fermented tempeh or miso are your best bets.

✔ Refer to the "Menopause" section in this chapter for more on soy prod-ucts and how they can mimic the effects of estrogen.

Be in the know about goitrogen veggies

Since childhood, you've always been told to eat your veggies — but what if I told you that eating too much of them may actually impact your thyroid function? Most of the studies that confirm this have been conducted in rats, so more research is needed for humans. The vegetables that have caused decreased production of thyroid hormone in rats are from the *Brassica* family, and they contain compounds called isothiocyanates which may act the same way as soy isoflavones. These veggies include:

- ✔ Cabbage
- ✔ Broccoli
- ✔ Cauliflower
- ✔ Brussels sprouts
- ✔ Kale

These veggies are also a rich source of glucosinolates, compounds which have anti-cancer benefits. In addition, they're excellent sources of vitamins, minerals, and fiber. When it comes to these foods, I'd include them cooked, steamed, or boiled, which help decrease the potential adverse effects. But don't eliminate them completely from your metabolism-boosting diet.

When to keep an eye on iodine

Getting enough iodine through your diet is important for your thyroid to churn out those hormones and to prevent too much of any food, such as soy or *Brassica* vegetables, from having a real impact on your thyroid function. Iodine is found in the following foods and food products:

- ✔ Seafood and seaweed products
- ✔ Fruits and vegetables grown in iodine-rich soil
- ✔ Dairy products
- ✔ Iodized salt

You may be surprised to know that iodine deficiency isn't that rare, even though table salt began to be iodized in the 20th century for this reason. Many places around the world have soil that's deficient in iodine. For example, the area around the Great Lakes in the U.S. was called the goiter belt before salt was iodized. But even today, depending on where you live and the foods you eat, it's possible that you're not getting enough.

Do not take iodine supplements without consulting your physician — and before increasing it in your diet, get your levels checked. Too much iodine is toxic and can result in side effects such as burning in the gastrointestinal tract, vomiting, coma, and even hyperthyroidism and thyroid cancer. Most adults should stay below 900–1,100 micrograms of iodine per day.

Seek out selenium

A deficiency in the trace mineral selenium can impair your thyroid's ability to convert hormones into their active form. Because of this, too little selenium can actually exacerbate an iodine deficiency by making hormone production even more difficult. Selenium is used to make antioxidants and therefore is important for your immune function. It can potentially help prevent cancer and boost male fertility.

Similar to iodine, selenium deficiencies can occur in places where soil content of selenium is low. Incorporate more of these selenium-rich foods into your diet:

- ✔ Brazil nuts
- ✔ Shellfish
- ✔ Sunflower seeds
- ✔ Grains
- ✔ Eggs

Should you go gluten-free?

Gluten-free diets have been a trend for some time, promising weight loss and improved health. However, I'd never advise you try this type of diet without scientific cause. The only people who absolutely must avoid gluten products are those diagnosed with Celiac disease, an allergy to the protein gluten, which is found in wheat, rye, and barley. A gluten-free diet is also recommended for those with a gluten-sensitivity. Not staying on a gluten-free diet can result in digestive symptoms and being unable to absorb nutrients properly, as well as continuing to cause damage to your intestines.

Thyroid diseases like Hashimoto's and Grave's disease are also autoimmune disorders like Celiac disease, meaning your body attacks its own natural processes. A study published in *Digestive Diseases and Science* found a link between Celiac disease and Hashimoto's and Grave's disease, suggesting that undiagnosed Celiac may trigger a thyroid condition and vice versa.

The study found that after following a gluten-free diet, the antibodies that signal an autoimmune disorder decreased. However, before going on a gluten-free diet, check with your doctor to see whether these antibodies are even increased. Remember, many nutritious foods like whole grain contain gluten, so don't use this for a means of weight loss. View a gluten-free diet as a way to improve your body's immune response with a thyroid condition. To follow a gluten-free diet, you need to avoid the following:

- ✔ Grains containing wheat, rye, and barley.
- ✔ Oats that are contaminated with gluten from other grains produced in the same facility.
- ✔ Any foods containing derivatives of those products, such as flours and processed foods with wheat, thickeners, malt flavoring, and modified food starch.

For more on how to go gluten-free the healthy way, check out *Living Gluten-Free For Dummies* (Wiley, 2010).

As with iodine, it's possible to have too much selenium, so don't start taking supplements without checking with your doctor and limit intake to less than 400 micrograms per day, and don't eat more than two Brazil nuts per day.

Making sure you have the right amount of selenium and iodine is important to a healthy thyroid.

Presenting with PCOS

If you're dealing with polycystic ovarian syndrome (PCOS), you're in the company of roughly 1 out of every 15 women in the U.S. who have the condition. Your hormones become unbalanced, which can affect how you look and feel, your menstrual cycle, and your fertility. You have a greater risk of developing PCOS if another woman in your family also had small cysts on her ovaries. It's these cysts that cause the hormone imbalance.

Although it's not 100 percent clear why these cysts develop, what is clear is that your risk for diabetes is higher: about 50 percent of PCOS sufferers have diabetes or pre-diabetes. It's similar to metabolic syndrome in that you're at increased risk for heart attack, high blood pressure, high cholesterol, as well as anxiety and depression. Therefore, you need to be extra diligent about your diet and choosing nutritious foods — which can be a powerful prevention tool.

Homing in on PCOS hormones

The hormonal changes you experience with PCOS have everything to do with the fact that these cysts impair the regular functions of your ovaries:

- ✔ You produce more androgens such as testosterone, the male sex hormone. Ovulation is impaired, so you may have abnormal menstrual cycles as well as difficulty with fertility. Too much male hormone also causes acne and hirsutism, or unwanted facial and body hair.

- ✔ You have difficulty processing insulin. When your blood sugar levels are high, and insulin isn't able to clear it out like it's supposed to, your pancreas works harder and harder to pump out more insulin to control your blood sugar levels. Over time, your cells become less and less sensitive to insulin, resulting in insulin resistance with an increased risk for diabetes. Being unable to use glucose for energy, your body then stores it as fat.

✔ Too much insulin and androgen leads to accumulating more abdominal, or visceral, fat around your organs. You can be at a healthy weight but still have too much of this fat, which puts you at increased risk for metabolic disease. But this isn't the norm — about 80 percent of women with PCOS are overweight or obese.

✔ Your hunger hormone, ghrelin, could be disregulated. This means that you may be more hungry and less able to sense your satiety, or fullness.

Research shows that a combination of diet and prescribed medication, such as oral hypoglycemic agents used for diabetes, can help regulate your menstrual cycles, fertility, and overall health. The most effective diet for PCOS focuses on aspects to improve your insulin sensitivity and reduce your weight.

If you're a smoker with PCOS, you need to strongly consider quitting once and for all. A study published in the journal of *Gynecological Endocrinology* found that women with PCOS who smoked had

✔ Higher blood lipids like cholesterol and triglycerides.

✔ Lower prolactin levels correlating to decreased fertility.

✔ More of the stress hormone cortisol secreted from the adrenal glands. This can cause increased blood pressure, blood glucose, a decrease in thyroid function, and increased abdominal fat storage.

Nicotine is certainly addictive, but just as you can take steps to change your diet, make taking steps to quit cigarettes a priority as well. For more information on why and how to kick the habit, see my free online article "Taking Care to Change Your Lifestyle" at www.dummies.com/extras/boosting yourmetabolism.

Making your diet PCOS-friendly

Although you've got to cut calories for weight loss, making that strategy effective for PCOS means not cutting out too many and packing the most nutrition you can into the calories you do eat. To lose weight at a steady rate, you need to reduce about 500 calories from your diet (or increase exercise to burn 500, or do a mixture of both) per day — without dipping below 1,200 calories, which can slow your metabolism. But what should comprise the calories you do take in when you have PCOS?

The goals of nutrition therapy with PCOS are weight loss if you're overweight, reducing your body fat percentage (if you're over 31 percent body fat), optimizing blood glucose control, and balancing out your hormones overall. There's overlap between hypothyroid and diabetes, so check out that

section of this chapter as well to help devise what your individual meal plan can look like. Following a consistent carbohydrate diet and eating every 4–5 hours helps create a balance among your blood glucose, hormones, and appetite.

When restricting your diet and getting nutritious foods, especially with a hormone-disrupting condition like PCOS, you need to make sure you're satisfied with the foods that you eat. If you feel hungry or deprived, something's got to give. You're probably not feeding yourself properly and you won't be able to sustain that in the long run. For a well-rounded diet with PCOS, focus on getting enough:

Fiber

Fiber helps buffer the impact that carbohydrates have on your blood glucose levels. That's because fiber takes longer to be digested and isn't quickly absorbed like refined carbohydrates, which cause rapid peaks and drops in blood glucose. Because of the extra time for digestion, fiber helps keep you fuller longer. Aim for about 25–40 grams per day from whole grains, fruits, vegetables, and legumes.

Go slow with adding more fiber into your diet. Too much, and you'll have stomach issues like constipation and bloating — especially if you're not matching the fiber increase with more water in your diet. Add about 5 grams of fiber per day and stay at that level for about a week or until you feel used to it and then build on that until you're at your goal.

Foods high in fiber tend to also be rich in other nutrients that can improve blood glucose as well as reduce your risk for heart disease with PCOS. For example, magnesium and B vitamins are found in the nutrient-rich bran and germ of a whole grain, but when a grain is refined, these nutrients are removed. Check out the anatomy of a whole grain in Chapter 4 for more.

Magnesium

Women with PCOS have significantly lower levels of the mineral magnesium, so getting more through your diet may help the risk factors that come along with PCOS as well:

- ✔ Low magnesium is correlated with insulin resistance and increased blood pressure.
- ✔ Get more from foods like bran, spinach, Brazil nuts, almonds, sunflower and flaxseeds, and dark chocolate.

Vitamin B12

All the B vitamins function to help your body convert nutrients to energy, but lower levels of B12 have been observed specifically in women with PCOS. Because B12 is mainly found in animal products, if you're following a vegetarian or vegan diet, you may need a supplement:

- ✔ Low B12 is correlated with insulin resistance, obesity, and elevated homocysteine — an amino acid (non-protein) that is a strong risk factor for heart disease.
- ✔ Get B12 in your diet from sources like shellfish and seafood, eggs, low-fat milk, and fortified breakfast cereals.

Omega 3 fatty acids

Not only are omega-3 fatty acids beneficial to reducing inflammation and improving blood cholesterol levels, they're also even more relevant to PCOS:

- ✔ Omega-3 fatty acids may help lower the male sex hormone, decreasing unwanted side effects like facial hair.
- ✔ Research shows omega-3 can help you feel more satisfied by increasing your body's sensitivity to leptin, the hormone that tells you you're full.
- ✔ Get omega-3s from fatty fish, nuts (especially walnuts), seeds like flax and chia, and omega-3–fortified eggs.

Zinc

Zinc is a mineral that may also help increase circulating leptin to help you become more in tune with your physical hunger. Start off your meal with oysters, which are a great source of zinc, as well as whole grains and red meat.

Leptin decreases as your weight decreases and as you reduce the calories you're taking in, making it more difficult to keep your appetite in check. Getting lean protein at every meal, which contains nutrients like zinc, B vitamins, and omega-3 fatty acids, can help offset this change in your hormones — especially because your hunger hormone ghrelin may increase with PCOS. Lean proteins like seafood, lower-in-fat cuts of red meat and poultry, low-fat dairy, beans, and eggs are all good options for you.

Calcium and vitamin D

Most women with PCOS, and many who are infertile, are also deficient in vitamin D and calcium. The two go hand in hand. Calcium may improve insulin sensitivity and requires vitamin D for absorption, and they both are required for ovarian follicle development. If you can't get enough from food, there may be cause to take supplements. Here are some calcium and vitamin D facts:

✔ Calcium is found in low-fat dairy, green leafy vegetables like collards and spinach, almonds, and sardines. Or take a supplement with 1,000 milligrams per day. To find out the best supplemental calcium to take, see Chapter 5.

✔ Vitamin D is found in fortified milk, salmon, tuna, mackerel, sardines, eggs, sunshine (helps convert vitamin D to most active form), and shiitake and button mushrooms. Or take a supplement with 400 IU per day.

For more info on many of these boosting foods and nutrients, I go more in depth in Chapter 5. Also refer to Table 12-2 for the top ten foods to incorporate into your diet with PCOS.

Table 12-2	PCOS Power Foods
Food	*Power Nutrients*
Flaxseed	Omega-3 fatty acids, fiber, magnesium
Bran flakes	Fiber, magnesium, vitamin B12
Low-fat yogurt	Calcium, vitamin B12
Salmon	Omega-3 fatty acids, vitamin B12, vitamin D
Almonds	Fiber, calcium, magnesium
Eggs	Vitamin B12, vitamin D, omega-3 (if fortified)
Dark chocolate	Magnesium, zinc
Oysters	Zinc, calcium, vitamin B12, omega-3
Lean red meat	Vitamin B12, zinc
Spinach	Calcium, fiber, magnesium

Fight back against insulin resistance to reduce your risk of developing diabetes with PCOS:

✔ **Monitor your caffeine intake.** It's possible that too much caffeine can reduce insulin sensitivity by up to 15 percent, according to a study published in *Diabetes Care*. So if you typically pound several cups of coffee or diet soda, consider cutting back or avoiding caffeine completely.

✔ **Limit refined carbohydrates.** This isn't to say a piece of white bread can never pass your lips, but too much refined carbohydrates leads to more erratic blood glucose levels.

✔ **Don't forget about activity.** Exercise helps improve insulin sensitivity and boosts your weight loss overall. See Chapter 11 to get started on an exercise plan.

Making Peace with Menopause

Hot flashes, mood swings, trouble sleeping, decreased sex drive, and even weight gain — oh, the joys of menopause. Menopause, occurring between the ages of about 40 and 60 years of age, is a natural time in every woman's life when the ovaries stop making estrogen and progesterone, the hormones required for reproduction.

Menopause is a vital time in your life for good nutrition. If you've never cared about your health before, at menopause you may reconsider changing your diet and lifestyle to reduce those undesirable side effects, help thwart weight gain, and keep you aging gracefully.

Weight gain and a slower metabolic rate are common in menopause due to the natural aging process and fluctuations in estrogen. Also, an increase in testosterone is one reason for the decreased sex drive. Menopause is a clear sign that your body is changing, and women in menopause tend to

✔ Move less and eat more calories than needed.

✔ Experience an increase in abdominal fat.

✔ Lose muscle mass, which is more metabolically active tissue.

✔ Experience mood swings and depression because estrogen levels impact the amount of the feel-good chemical serotonin.

Whether to engage in hormone replacement therapy (HRT) is a personal decision between you and your doctor. Although HRT can reduce symptoms of menopause, it may also increase your risk for stroke and cancer.

You can't just blame your hormones and give up any hope of feeling good during this stage in your life. Poor eating habits can exacerbate the symptoms you experience. Nutritious foods and exercise help improve your mood and your metabolic rate. With menopause, these nutrients may help reduce side effects:

✔ Vitamins E and C are powerful antioxidants that can lessen hot flashes, reduce irritability and anxiety, and boost your energy levels.

✔ Vitamin E is routinely prescribed for menopausal patients in supplement form of 400–800 IU. You can also find it in vitamin E–rich foods like nuts, wheat germ, green leafy vegetables, and tropical fruits.

✔ Calcium and vitamin D are important to ward off osteoporosis because fluctuating estrogen decreases bone density. In menopause, aim for 1,200 milligrams of calcium per day. For more on foods containing calcium and vitamin D, see the earlier "PCOS" section.

✔ Soy isoflavones are phytoestrogens, so named because they can mimic estrogen and actually help reduce side effects like hot flashes. However, conflicting studies have also shown that taking too much of these may promote cancer growth. Instead of taking supplements, choose foods rich in soy like edamame, soy milk, soy nuts, miso, tofu, and tempeh.

✔ Complex carbohydrate and fiber help keep your energy levels high and your body satisfied. You may crave more carbohydrates and sweets when your serotonin drops. Many carbohydrates affect your tryptophan levels in the blood, a precursor for serotonin, so choosing high-fiber foods like whole grains can help stave off cravings, improve your health overall, and help with weight loss. These foods also help you get a good night's sleep, which can be difficult during menopause.

Fight the bloat! Many women experience bloating during menopause which may be eased by the following:

✔ **Decreasing salty foods:** Choose salt-free herbs and spices to flavor foods and watch your consumption of processed, prepared foods, cured meats and cheese. Check the sodium on all condiments. When out to eat, ask for sauces on the side to help control and reduce the amount, and never be ashamed to ask your waiter to request food be prepped sans salt.

✔ **Monitoring your alcohol intake:** Bloating is a common after-effect of alcohol, and alcohol is a trigger for hot flashes. Stick to one drink per day or less.

✔ **Don't skimp on water:** You may be tempted not to drink water because you feel that'll cause you to be more bloated. That's not necessarily the case — water can actually help flush out your system and keep you hydrated and your energy high.

If you've made changes with your diet outlined here and with foods from Chapter 5 but still aren't having any luck with weight loss or improvements in mood, ask yourself if you can be doing more in the exercise department. Often, that's the key to relax, improve sleep, and help give your metabolism a healthy boost.

Chapter 13

Staying on the Metabolism-Boosting Bandwagon

· ·

In This Chapter

▶ Learning how to overcome common weight-loss barriers

▶ Creating a balance to help you stay the course

▶ Influencing your loved ones to change unhealthy habits and have fun doing it

· ·

1 know how the story goes. You get motivated to make changes to your diet and lifestyle in preparation for a wedding, reunion, bathing suit season, as a New Year's resolution, or in response to seeing an unflattering photo of yourself. You go to the grocery store, stock up on healthy foods and books like this one, maybe even purchase a gym membership. You're planning for a complete overhaul of your diet.

The changes you make last for a week, a month, or even longer … before something happens that causes a hard stop. Either your motivation wavers, or you don't have the time or energy to devote to the cause, or you haven't been seeing results so you think "what's the point?" — or you're just sick and tired and bored of the foods you're eating, and going to the gym feels like torture.

I've heard the story time and time again, and always at the root, the moral of the story is that there's no such thing as a magic bullet that will get you where you want to be with your weight and health. The key to being successful at reaching your metabolism-boosting goals and making lifestyle changes is three-pronged:

✔ You have to be realistic.

✔ You have to plan ahead for both when you succeed and when you fail.

✔ You have to have the support of friends and family

This chapter shows you how to take those steps and reshape your thinking from quick-fix diet plan to long-term success.

Battling Roadblocks

Along your weight loss journey, you'll inevitably hit roadblocks. These are what you use as excuses to not forge ahead with your healthy plan. When you're stuck in stalled traffic, you make the most of it — or search for an alternate route to get to your destination. Think of your road to a healthier you in the same way; you'll have setbacks and barriers, such as lack of time, money, or energy. Staying optimistic and understanding the steps you can take to continue evolving help keep you going full steam ahead.

Getting past the "Monday diet" hurdle

Monday is the first day of the work week for most people and, therefore, the day that you may think of as a fresh start, especially after an indulgent or lazy weekend.

Not all excuses are to get out of doing something. Monday can be a great excuse to start make changes — you can prep over the weekend and have a healthier outlook for the week ahead. But, by prepping over the weekend, I don't mean pigging out in prep for a week of restrictive eating and boot camp exercising, like the "all or nothing" mentality I talk about in Chapter 4. I mean planning ahead by picking up items at the grocery store and deciding what you'll eat and how you'll exercise for the week.

Recently, a client who's a teacher told me that during the following summer she'd get back on track with healthy habits because she'd have more time. It turned out that during the summer she wanted to "enjoy herself" and didn't even think about the healthy steps she could take. She then let me know that the school year is an easier time to stick with it since she has more structure in place.

It's more realistic to figure out how you can make changes to your diet and fit in exercise during what your life looks like most of the time. You'll need to regularly make tweaks as your routine changes. Putting off making changes is pointless, because if you can't make them today, why do you think you'll act on them later on? There's no day like today, even if it's not a Monday.

Making time for healthy habits

People who make time for exercise and healthy eating habits don't magically have more hours in the day than you do. Not having enough time is one of the top excuses for not making lifestyle changes. Think about my schoolteacher client: Even when she did have time, she didn't use it to reaching her goals. And although making lifestyle changes certainly isn't easy, making excuses doesn't get you anywhere. Instead, start thinking positively about where you can fit in a change here and there in your day. If you truly want to make changes, with the following tips, you'll find a way to make it work for you.

Redefining how you picture exercise and a balanced diet can help you make time for healthy habits. Set aside the overhaul for a second and think about smaller steps you can take.

Healthy eating doesn't have to mean slaving over the stove for hours and having perfectly planned meals. Instead, define it as the following:

- Stocking your kitchen with nutritious foods, snacks, and frozen, ready-to-cook ingredients like fruits, vegetables, and lean protein sources. If you can't get to the grocery store, order groceries online or give your list to a family member. You can repay the favor another time.

- Being savvy when dining out. Just because you don't have time to cook doesn't mean you can't make healthy decisions at a restaurant or when you order in. Chapter 14 has tips on how to eat healthy on-the-go in any situation.

- If you do have time to cook once per week, make multiple batches of your meals; bring leftovers for lunch or freeze for other meals later in the week.

- Making one food swap at a time, such as fat-free milk instead of 2 percent milk in your cereal, drinking seltzer or water instead of soda, or choosing whole-wheat bread instead of white bread for your sandwiches. Every change counts.

- Spending 20 minutes on Sunday creating a tentative food plan for the week ahead. You can try to make it an activity with your family so that you'll come up with meals you'll all enjoy. Writing out a list can be very helpful for your reference, even if you're not able to stick to it all of the time. Use this list to decide what groceries you need.

Getting exercise doesn't have to mean having a sweat-fest at the gym. Start smaller with the following:

- Walking during lunch break or taking the stairs at the office instead of the elevator.

- Waking up 20 minutes earlier to do an exercise DVD in your home.

- Walking around the house while on the phone, or doing squats in place.

✔ Marching in place during commercials when watching television, or doing crunches, or better yet, watching your favorite show while on the treadmill or stationary bicycle.

✔ Dividing a longer workout into two mini-workouts throughout the day.

Don't go it alone. Saying you don't have time is easy if you're only accountable to yourself. If you have a friend or family member also trying to change their lifestyle, swap meal ideas, go out to eat and split an entrée, and make a plan to take an exercise class together. It helps when you can get some fun out of the changes you're making, so it doesn't seem like a total drag on your lifestyle. More on the power of support later in this chapter.

Minding your wallet and waistline

You don't have to blow your budget on a healthy lifestyle. "Eating healthy is too expensive and not worth it" is an excuse I often hear. You may have uttered these words if you've been on a specific diet plan where you need to purchase special meals or use recipes with exotic or hard-to-find foods.

Getting your grocery budget down while adding healthy items doesn't happen overnight. It requires planning and trial and error. According to the USDA, a budget of $40 per week can get one adult to meet all nutrient requirements and for a family of four, $145 per week can do the trick. Prices are based on averages in the United States, so depending on where you live, it may be more or less. To meet those marks, you have to be thrifty.

These swaps not only help your wallet but also your waistline when it comes to getting the most nutritional bang for your buck:

✔ Choose frozen fruits and vegetables for a variety of produce all year round. Save $0.25 per ounce.

✔ Choose frozen, lean meats like bottom round roast in bulk. Save $1.50 per pound.

✔ Go vegetarian once a week and choose cheaper sources of protein like dried peas or beans, peanut butter, and eggs. Save $0.40 per ounce.

✔ Keep nonfat dry milk on hand and buy low-fat milk and yogurt in the largest containers you can, though make sure they get used before expiring. Save $1 per cup.

✔ Choose day-old whole-wheat breads and freeze any fresh bread that you can't use immediately. Save at least $1 per loaf.

✔ Choose steel-cut oats and regular brown rice instead of instant varieties. Save $0.15 per ounce.

Convenience foods — meaning pre-cut, pre-washed, pre-packaged — cost more due to cost of labor. If you truly don't have time to cut your own fruits and veggies, and this is worth the cost for you, then go for it in the name of healthy eating. See my free online article "Setting Up Your Kitchen for Success" at www.dummies.com/extras/boostingyourmetabolism/ for more cost-cutting tips for the grocery store.

Dining out is another story. Cooking at home will help you save the most money, but isn't always practical. How to save money when eating out:

- ✔ **Have happy hour at home.** If you plan to have an alcoholic drink, do it at home before heading out (if you're not driving) or when you get home. Restaurants hike up the price of their liquor, and you may succumb to fancy cocktails which add up calorically and financially.

- ✔ **Take advantage of technology.** Popular coupon sites like Groupon or checking in on Foursquare on your smart phone may bring up deals at your favorite dining establishments or can help you search places in the area to go with discounts and special deals.

- ✔ **Do your research.** Look at menus ahead of time to check the cost and put together a healthy meal within your budget. Most restaurant menus are available online.

- ✔ **Practice portion control.** By splitting entrees with a buddy and taking a doggy bag home, you'll be watching your waistline and your wallet.

You may be spending your money frivolously in the name of a smaller waistline. Remember, there's no such thing as a magic bullet, so don't succumb to these traps from the billion-dollar weight loss industry:

- ✔ Fancy marketing for foods or vitamins — generic or regular versions are often just as effective.

- ✔ Specialty weight-loss supplements or drugs, "diet plan" food products, or meal replacements.

- ✔ Gym memberships that you don't use (if you use it and it motivates you to exercise, that's another thing). You can get a great workout at home, without equipment; I outline a plan for you to do so in Chapter 11.

Being real with yourself

I'd like to interrupt this chapter to remind you that you can't do everything all at once. A complete overhaul of your lifestyle all at once isn't going to last in the long term. If you've done fad or restrictive diets in the past, you may have noticed that although they promise quick results, often you end up back where you started. Yet time and time again, I see people going back to them. If it didn't work then, why would it work now?

You need to be realistic with your weight-loss goals and with the strategies you'll use to get to those goals. If you believe one of the following statements, go back and read Chapter 4 to assess your readiness for lifestyle change:

- ✔ I need to avoid all my favorite foods to lose weight.

- ✔ I must work out for an hour every day to burn enough calories.

- ✔ I will only eat food I prepare because I don't know what goes into restaurant meals.

- ✔ I can't go out with my friends to eat anymore.

- ✔ I'll stop drinking alcohol forever.

These statements probably aren't realistic and you're setting yourself up for failure by making them when they can't be sustained. If you're real with yourself, come up with a list of changes that you know you can really work, such as making smaller swaps. If you can't always achieve those goals, there's no such thing as undoing all the positive change you've made. Every experience is a way to learn how to improve when you're in that situation again.

You know you've made it far toward a lifestyle change when you've mastered dining out. Many social situations revolve around food, and it's hard to eat perfectly when you don't necessarily have input into the food that's being served or ordered for you. This becomes a major issue for many around holiday season. Being real with yourself means the following:

- ✔ **Not saying:** "I'll never dine out" or "I'll always eat before an event and just go to socialize."

- ✔ **Saying:** "I'll limit the times per week I dine out" or "I'll make healthier choices when at parties."

For advice on how to dine out or make the best decisions in any situation when on the go, see Chapter 14.

Forgetting about willpower

Did you gasp when reading that heading? What would you say if I told you willpower is a myth — that it's just an excuse for you not to take control of your own destiny. Willpower is another major barrier that builds up brick by brick into a reason for not reaching your goals.

One of the damaging effects the belief that you "just don't have the willpower" can have is to make you think that you're just not good enough. It makes you feel shameful — as though there's something wrong with you that you can't say no to a slice of cake, that you can't stay motivated at the gym for longer than five minutes, or that you hit up the vending machine every day. Don't forget about the external factors at play:

✔ Your friend saying, "You only live once — eat cake!" Let friends know you're trying hard to cut down on sweets and you'd truly appreciate their support.

✔ The fact that you're not sure how to use most of the equipment at the gym. Try an exercise class that you find fun and entertaining. Or request assistance from a gym staff member on the machines you'd like to learn.

✔ You're going too many hours between meals and you're hungry. Of course you're looking for something to eat, and vending machines don't typically have the best options. Pack yourself a nutritious snack to plan ahead for those long stretches.

Instead of this mythical "willpower," what you need is motivation to make changes in your life. And you're just not going to be motivated by a flip of a switch — like suddenly having willpower or not. You're motivated by both external and internal factors, and you *stay* motivated by having a plan to set yourself up for success and regularly reminding yourself of your goals.

If you don't feel like you have any structure in your life, or you have an erratic work schedule or hectic family life, you can take steps towards the end goal. Create a timeline and plan week by week the changes you'll make, and when you're tempted to stray, ask yourself, is doing this going to help me get to my goal? Think about how hard you're working and the personal gift of good health you're giving yourself by staying the course. You may come to the conclusion that indulging in that temptation isn't worth it to you after all. That's the secret to overcoming the willpower monster.

Mastering How To "Cheat"

For you to reach your goals, you've got to learn how to give in a little — otherwise, you'll give in a lot when your resolve is low and you're faced with temptation. Not being able to achieve a balance may be the reason you aren't able to lose weight. I use the word *cheat* because it's a known word in this regard. But as much as you're able, don't think of it as doing something dishonest; it's just a natural part of your lifestyle change.

This may sound completely counterintuitive to you. It's true that if you want to lose weight and boost your metabolism, you need to choose nutritious foods, stay within your calorie needs, and get plenty of activity. But by allowing yourself to indulge occasionally, you won't feel deprived and you'll be able to stick to those positive life-changing habits most of the time. Otherwise, you'll ride the rollercoaster of being "good" and "bad" with your "diet" all throughout your life.

How much can you indulge before it's considered excessive? That's the million dollar question! It's a fine line to walk, which is why many fall to one side or the other. In this chapter, I provide you with the best strategies for balance with your diet so you can boost your metabolism and still enjoy life.

Why taking a break is great

Taking a break really works on many levels, both mentally and physically. If you have the mentality that you're not going to see results unless you're "perfect" with eating and exercise, listen up! There's no such thing as perfect when it comes to your eating. It doesn't exist. Because if you're too restrictive, it backfires — either you can't sustain it or it isn't healthy for your body, and that sure doesn't sound too perfect to me.

When you believe in an ideal world of perfect eating, you tend to ignore your physical hunger cues. Instead of eating when you're hungry and stopping when you're full, you eat based on a limited meal plan which may not be satisfying. The more you ignore what your body is telling you, the harder it is to pay attention to these physical cues, so emotions are more likely to take over. For more about your body on a diet, see Chapter 1.

However, you *are* making changes to how you're eating and the calories you're taking in, so mentally you make an adjustment. Also, you're more aware of the food that's going into your body, which takes more brainpower, and as you begin to lose weight, your metabolism does change.

So, the good news is that my advice is to take a break from making sure every morsel that goes into your mouth is nutritious and counting every calorie. Having a balance helps you

✔ Say goodbye to side effects of restriction such as low energy, rocky mood, constant thoughts about food and cravings, and increased tendency to overeat or emotionally eat. Allowing yourself to indulge in moderation helps reduce these urges and helps you keep your sanity.

✔ Say goodbye to plateaus with your weight. As you lose weight, your leptin levels and thyroid hormones drop, along with your ability to sense satiety and your metabolic rate. That's why the last pounds are the hardest to lose. Taking controlled breaks encourages increases in these hormones to counteract the effect they have on your halted weight loss.

✔ Say hello to a boosted metabolic rate and a lifestyle change. Instead of being sucked into quick fixes and extreme dieting methods, you'll be able to create a balance so that you can sustain new healthy behaviors for the long run.

Following the 80/20 rule

Although I'm against strict food rules, the 80/20 rule is one made for cheating! It's not exactly your Get Out of Jail Free card, because remember: Balance is key here.

The core of 80/20 is this: Make 4 out of 5 choices a healthy one. That means 80 percent of the time you make nutritious choices, and 20 percent of the time you aren't so strict with what you eat. Twenty percent of the time you can indulge in dining out, eat at a party or work event, consume alcohol or metabolism-busting foods like sodium, refined carbohydrate, or saturated fats.

You can also use the 80/20 rule in other helpful ways:

- ✔ Only eat 80 percent of your plate when dining out to help control portions. This helps you remember that having the entire plate may be way too much (although, of course, plate sizes and contents vary). Quit your membership in the Clean Plate Club, where you always feel like you have to finish every last item on your plate.

- ✔ Stop when you're 80 percent full, so you don't get overstuffed. In other words, on a scale from 0–10, where 0 is you feel ravenous and 10 is uncomfortably full, you should stop eating when you're a 7 or 8.

- ✔ Exercise 80 percent of days in the week or at least get some sort of activity or movement in at least 5 days per week.

In some cases, 20 percent may be too much. If your blood glucose levels are uncontrolled, I don't encourage that you consume 20 percent of your calories in soda and gummy bears. Also, if you have a food allergy like Celiac disease, 20 percent can't go toward foods containing gluten, because that can be damaging to your health.

You may need to be a bit more diligent with your diet depending on your individual condition. But don't think just because you've tried everything to lose weight and haven't that you have zero margin for enjoying the foods you love in moderation. Aim for at least 10 percent of your calories from treats. So, if you're following a 1,600 calorie diet, have between 100–200 calories from your favorite fun food per day to help keep you interested in a healthy eating plan.

Planning how to "cheat"

There may be some foods you feel like you need to abstain from completely because they're "trigger" foods for you, meaning they prompt you to overeat. But unless you have a food allergy, you can learn how to include every type of food within your calorie budget without sabotaging your health. It takes time to master the art of balance, but once you do, you'll be able to lose the guilt and savor the foods you love in a new way.

Letting foods out of jail can be very liberating. By telling yourself that it's okay to have something you've viewed as "forbidden" in the past, your idealization of the food diminishes, and you're less likely to crave and feel shame surrounding it. I've seen this in action with many clients who never thought they could let their forbidden foods out of jail.

Why you shouldn't make it a "cheat" weekend

It may be much easier for you to stick to healthy habits during the week when you have a routine and structure based on your work schedule. But on the weekend, you may go out to dinner, go to the movies, and attend birthday parties and events that impact what you eat and drink. Planning to indulge all weekend long and being diligent with your diet during the week may sound like a good idea to you, but it's not, and here's why:

✔ Weekend splurges propagate the *all or nothing* mentality that hurts your best efforts.

✔ If you plot to be indulgent on the weekend, you may make the less healthy choice even if you're not really in the mood for it or you may tell yourself "I was good all week, I deserve this." Using food as a reward for being healthy can hurt you in the long run, making you more prone to emotional eating.

✔ Planning to be off of healthy habits for two whole days can get out of control. Although it doesn't completely undo all your good efforts during the week, it makes it more and more difficult for you to lose weight and feel your best.

Instead, try to make the weekend as much as possible like a weekday:

✔ Start the day off with a balanced breakfast no matter what time you wake up, and eat a meal or snack every 4–5 hours after that.

✔ Use extra free time on the weekend as an excuse to schedule activity.

✔ Try placing limits like sticking to one alcoholic drink each day of the weekend or only one meal of dining out whenever possible.

✔ Just because you have a party or special event doesn't mean you need to eat all the treats available to you there. Pay attention to your physical hunger cues and ask yourself what is really worth it to you.

A study published in the *International Journal of Obesity* found that those who kept a consistent diet throughout the week instead of restricting during the week and eating more on weekends were 1.5 times more likely to keep the weight off.

Certain beliefs about foods have been drilled into your head for years and years by the media, friends, and family. So it may be hard to embrace that carbohydrates aren't necessarily "fattening" or that you're allowed to eat after 8 p.m. or you can have a serving of ice cream without disrupting your healthy meal plan. It can be powerful to remind yourself that it's not the last time you're ever going to eat ice cream. You can have it again tomorrow if it fits into your calorie intake and that's what you choose to have.

Before going out and stocking up on foods you plan to "cheat" with, follow these guidelines:

✔ Don't make the entire day or meal a "cheat" unless you have no other option. You can always start off with a balanced breakfast, have a high-fiber snack, make time for exercise, or pair your meal with a serving of vegetables to have a balance.

✔ Don't keep jumbo-sized packages of treats in your house, especially if you have a history of being unable to "eat just one."

✔ Don't let your cravings decide when you'll cheat. This can lead you to overeating in an uncontrolled environment.

✔ Do have a plan when going out to parties or restaurants where you know you'll be exposed to the foods you crave.

✔ Do choose pre-packaged single-serving portions of your cheat foods while on-the-go or pair them with a food that's nutrient dense so you won't be tempted to buy a second pack. If you don't want to spend the premium price for single-serve packages, an alternative is to portion your food out ahead of time. For example, take two cookies out of a package and put one away before eating. It makes it harder to have more, and if you do, it will be a more conscious choice.

✔ Do eat slowly and savor every single bite. You're meant to enjoy it after all. And remember, it takes about 20 minutes for your stomach to tell your brain you're full. Always keep paying attention to your physical hunger cues instead of giving yourself a license to overeat just because you're enjoying one serving of this food.

✔ Do indulge with friends and family if they're supportive and can help you stay accountable for how much you "cheat."

There's no one-size-fits-all approach to including less-than-nutritious foods in your metabolism-boosting plan. Here are some tips:

✔ You may know that you have a party to attend. Plan ahead for that event by being diligent with your meals beforehand. Navigate your party with tips from Chapter 14.

✔ You may want a decadent dessert once per week, so the rest of the week, choose fruit for dessert. Also, before you dig in, have a meal of lean protein and vegetables.

✔ You may let yourself have a treat or fun food every day in a small portion size to help ward off cravings — such as chocolate chips in your Greek yogurt or an ounce of cheese with whole-wheat crackers as a snack.

✔ You may be able to fly by the seat of your pants and have a bite here and there without making an entire meal, snack, or dessert out of it. But this is something you achieve when you've already practiced mindful eating and are really in tune with your hunger and fullness. An example would be picking a few French fries off your friend's plate at lunch or having a few bites of cake at a birthday party.

No matter how you "cheat," the most important thing is being real with yourself. Only you know your own limits regarding how well you're able to control your portions with your cravings. For tips on how to manage food cravings, see Chapter 16.

Getting Back on Track

In other aspects of your life — besides weight and health — things don't always go as planned, right? Maybe your goal is to be promoted to manager at your job or get married by a certain age and start a family. But another candidate gets the position, or you didn't find the right person. Do you stop going to work or stop dating and just give up hope because you didn't get what you wanted? No.

It's never too late to get right back on a metabolism-boosting track, no matter how many times you've tried and failed.

Acknowledging that success isn't a straight line and that you need to learn from your mistakes is a part of the process. That's why I like to think of every experience as just that — a way to learn and improve upon for next time. You can't undo the progress you've made. Each experience you have better equips you to handle a situation the next time. Eventually, healthy habits become second nature to you. The strategies in this section can help you do just that.

Planning your meals ahead

Once you have a goal in mind, one of the most effective ways to stay motivated is to plan ahead. Setting out a schedule for yourself and actually sticking to it is empowering.

It seems like a small thing, but instead of measuring your progress only by your weight, measure it by other accomplishments, like sticking to your meal plan or making time for exercise. This will help you get out of the mindset that you need to see results in the form of weight loss to keep you going.

Everyone's plan will be unique, based on food preferences, calorie needs, activity level, and many other factors. As you sit down to create a plan that will be realistic for you, keep these factors in mind:

- ✔ **Surveying your schedule:** When are you at work and when will you have downtime to go food shopping or cook? Do you have a date night planned, and where are you dining? Take a look at your schedule and see when you can fit in time for exercise.

- ✔ **Writing it out:** Writing down what you're eating and when can be very helpful for reminding yourself of your plan and keeping you accountable. Place a checkmark next to when you stuck to it and an X next to where you weren't so successful. Think about what happened in that moment and how you can improve next time.

✔ **Making swaps:** When you know you'll be in a difficult situation, how can you make a healthy swap? Is there an alternative option, like sneaking a protein bar into the movie theater instead of buying a jumbo box of candy? Or can you make a swap in a family recipe to healthify the dish, such as replacing sour cream with low-fat yogurt? Once you have your meals and activities mapped out, you can write notes about the best choices to make.

✔ **Don't do it alone:** Work on your meal plan with family or friends to help you stay accountable and incorporate the plan in with family meals and social events. Let as many people as you feel comfortable with know about the fact you're trying to get back on track. That way, you'll have more support in your corner when faced with hard decisions.

Use a blank schedule to write out all your meals and food-related activities for the week ahead. The sample meal plans in Chapter 6 can get you started. Table 13-1 gives you an idea of what your tool can look like.

Table 13-1	Meal Planning Tool						
	Sunday	*Monday*	*Tuesday*	*Wednesday*	*Thursday*	*Friday*	*Saturday*
Breakfast							
Lunch							
Dinner							
Snack							
Exercise							
Activity							

The activity row helps you plan out when you'll go grocery shopping and when you can pre-cook or prepare foods during the week. Use your weekly meal planner when you go grocery shopping to save time and money, because you'll only be purchasing items you plan to use that week.

Doing the next right thing

Also known as planning ahead for failure, if you eat an extra serving or indulged in a food that is out of your caloric budget, it doesn't mean the whole day has to be a bust. For many people, the belief that their "diet will start tomorrow" is the biggest instigator of falling off the bandwagon and being unable to get back on. You make one excuse after another about why you can't make the better decision in that instant, even if the opportunity is available to you.

Recently, Hurricane Sandy hit the New York tri-state area, and many of us were hunkered down without much food or water. Options for food were whatever you had stocked or supplied by the Red Cross, and maybe a pizza place in your neighborhood was open. Fresh fruits, vegetables, dairy, and other perishable goods were few and far between. After the storm had passed and power was restored, one friend joked that she had gained the "Sandy Seven" and that she really needed to get back on the healthy eating bandwagon.

In this case, there was no option but to sustain yourself with the foods available. But most of the time, you do have a choice, and the availability at your fingertips to do the *next* right thing. You don't have to wait until a proverbial storm or stressful situation or slip-up is way behind you to get back on track. Look forward at what you can do next, the next time you make a decision about food or activity.

Doing the *next* right thing means the following:

✔ After an indulgent night out, wake up and have a regular, balanced breakfast the next morning instead of skipping because you still feel full or bloated.

✔ If your coworker brings in cookies for your team in the morning, think about whether you're really hungry before having one. If you do, stick to your meal plan the rest of the day.

✔ If you find that you only have 30 minutes at the gym instead of an hour, do a 30-minute workout instead of forgoing the opportunity completely.

✔ If you're having a glass of alcohol with dinner, skip the bread basket and dessert.

These are just examples of how you don't need to picture your whole day as ruined and use that as an excuse to finish all the ice cream in the freezer just because something doesn't go as planned. Get back on track faster than waiting until the next day, next week, or next month to stick to your impossibly "perfect" plan — because a small blip may throw you off then, too.

When you can be too mindful

Being aware of what you're eating is important, but being hyperaware can make you overwhelmed and make it harder to get back on track. If your eating plan gives you anxiety either about whether or not you're making the right choice, or if you're stressed in social situations (or you avoid them) because of the food available, it's time to take a step back. When eating healthy interferes with your mental health, it's not a way to live.

Feeling shame or guilt about your food choices is counterproductive. Research shows that people who feel negative about their bodies and food choices are more likely to sabotage their healthy habits.

Orthorexia nervosa is a term coined by Steven Bratman, M.D. (a specialist in alternative medicine) to describe those who are very rigid about their choices and will only eat "clean" or nutritious foods so that they feel "pure." It's not a diagnosis or clinical term, but these are people who will go to extreme lengths to avoid any type of metabolism-buster like excess fat, sodium, or sugar — and they never eat out, preparing every food they consume from scratch to be sure about its contents.

Being "perfect" with healthy habits isn't the answer for getting back on track. In fact, it can have the opposite effect:

✔ It can border on obsessive compulsive behavior and cause you to isolate yourself and look down upon other's health practices.

✔ If you cut out certain food groups or are extremely rigid, you may miss out on valuable nutrients that do boost your metabolism.

✔ Being stressed all the time affects your hormones, can increase fat storage, and slow your metabolic rate. In fact, people who fall under this term aren't typically a low body weight.

If this sounds like you, seek the help of a mental professional to help you create more of a balance in your life.

Building support outside the home

Weight loss is more successful with support, plain and simple. I can rattle off statistics about people using online communities or in-person meetups being more likely to reach and maintain their health goals. The reasons speak for themselves. If you have a support group, friends, or a professional to confide in, the following things happen:

✔ You stay accountable for your healthy behaviors.

✔ You can share stories and see what has worked for others to stick to a plan.

✔ You recognize you aren't alone and have someone to turn to when discouraged to help you stay the course.

Everyone has different needs when it comes to support and various resources available to them. Table 13-2 outlines basic ways you can team up with people outside the home so you're more likely to stay on track (the next section covers support within your home).

Table 13-2	Support Outside the Home
Type	*What you'll get*
Online communities	An anonymous way to connect whenever you have the time
In-person weight-loss groups	Accountability with partners, activities like weigh-ins
Religious support groups	A way to mesh your spirituality with your health goals
Registered dietitian	A professional to be your "diet detective" who can provide insight and education about food and your health
Mental health counselor	A professional to talk to about how you may use food for reasons other than hunger and who can help you learn tools to change

Building Healthy Habits At Home

Your values about food, nutrition, and health emanate from home. They're formed by your childhood, your experiences throughout life, and how you raise your children moving forward. Within the first few years of life, children can pick up on parents' eating behaviors, thoughts, and cultural practices around food, which shapes how they eat and potentially their weight.

Unfortunately, home can be a place that sabotages your efforts if you have junk foods around for your spouse or kids. It's difficult to motivate others to see your point of view or give up keeping foods in the house they love or support you to make nutritious meals. This section talks about how to garner your family's support to get on the metabolism-boosting bandwagon with you. When that happens, you're much more likely to stay on as well.

Surrounding the kitchen table

The kitchen is often the watering hole of the house. In my home, it's where my family gathers even when we're not eating or even if there are snacks out in the living room where the television is. There's just something special about a kitchen table. It's where family communication happens and bonds form.

According to a review of research out of Rutgers University, when families eat together, they're more likely to get fiber from fruits and vegetables and get metabolism-boosting vitamins and minerals like calcium. Children from families who spend more time together around the kitchen table are more likely to have a lower BMI, show fewer signs of depression, and do better in school.

Sadly, families aren't eating together enough. Researchers found that much of the budget for food is spent outside of the home dining out. Although you can make healthy decisions when eating out, typically it's associated with more sodium, saturated fat, and excess calories overall.

It's challenging to make time to sit down and eat together because of conflicting work schedules, extracurricular activities, sports practices, and so on. But with a bit of thought you can make the best out of any situation. Here are some tips:

- **Family meals aren't just for dinner.** If you can take 20 minutes to sit down for breakfast, you can get your bonding time in first thing, and it's a great teaching opportunity about the importance of a balanced breakfast.

- **Get your family involved in meal prep.** Even if everyone can't sit down to the table, set aside a time for healthy cooking lessons with your kids. When children are involved in creating a meal, it's more exciting for them to eat it.

- **Eat with whoever is home.** Even if everyone can't sit down, it doesn't mean you can't have a family meal. When I was growing up, my father worked nights, and my brothers were older or out of the house, but my mom and I would eat together at home almost every weeknight.

- **Turn off the television and smart phones.** Whatever your family interaction around healthy habits looks like, TVs and phones disrupt the discussion. Make watching television around the kitchen table a special occasion, not the norm. Instead, ask about each other's day and hash out concerns going on at school or work.

Family meal time at home isn't only for getting a healthy meal in you. It's for decompressing after a busy day, creating a comfortable, stable, supportive home environment, teaching your children manners, and even saving money in the process.

Sure, it may be easier to order pizza or Chinese food or go to the drive-through, but family meal times don't have to be complicated. And actually, no matter what you eat, it still counts as family bonding time. If you never eat as a group, start with once or twice per week for a family meal time and build up from there. If you stock your kitchen with metabolism-boosting foods, healthy eating can be not only manageable but enjoyable.

Making meal time a family affair doesn't have to mean grilled chicken and steamed green veggies every night. If you're the one cooking, try Table 13-3's swaps in classic family favorite recipes to lighten up dishes without compromising on taste.

Table 13-3	Recipe swaps for family favorites	
Instead of...	*Use...*	*In recipes like...*
Ground beef	Lean ground turkey or bison	Meatloaf, chili, and meatballs
Bread crumbs	Crushed oats or quinoa, ground nuts or seeds	Chicken cutlets, nuggets, fish cakes, anything breaded
Whole milk/cheese	Low fat milk, part skim cheese	Mac and cheese, burritos, mashed potatoes, homemade pizza
Sour cream	Low fat Greek yogurt	Atop baked potato/Mexican dishes, in creamy soups
Too many noodles	Shredded spaghetti squash, zucchini, carrots	Any pasta main or side dish
Butter	Pureed fruit like canned pumpkin, avocado	Cakes, cookies, pies, muffins

Making food fun for kids

If you have a picky eater on your hands, mealtime is anything but fun. You're running around trying to figure out what foods your kids will actually eat while trying to prepare nutritious meals for yourself — it can be exhausting and affect what's on your plate. Sometimes, kids just need a little bit of creativity with their meals — instead of looking down at a boring plate of meat, baked potato, and Brussels sprouts — to get them excited about trying new foods.

Never push any food on your child — they'll be more likely to turn their nose up. Instead offer a variety of foods and offer them more than once. Just because you were turned down once doesn't mean your child won't try it ever again if presented in a different way or paired with a food you know they love.

Because you have to compete with ads for sugary beverages and snack foods with your child's favorite cartoon characters on them, get inspired to make healthy food fun by creating an activity out of it. Let your children come help you pick groceries at the store. Think about starting a garden or try container gardening in your backyard or patio. Seeing the vegetables and herbs grow from the ground may give your kids (and you) a sense of pride and a greater appreciation of what they're eating.

In the kitchen, make arts and craft with food. It'll get messy and take longer than it would if you put something together quickly, but it's worth it to get your kids interested about healthy items so that your diet won't suffer from too many snack foods in the house. Here are some ideas:

- **Revamp the classic ants on a log.** In addition to peanut butter spread on celery sticks with raisins atop, get creative with various ingredients so your kids can pick and choose how to make this old-time favorite. Try bases like apples, watermelon, pineapple, carrots, jicama, or cucumbers cut into slices. Top with a spoonful of yogurt, spreadable cheese, or guacamole. Add "ants" like dark chocolate chips, seeds, nuts, or beans.

- **Make your own mini pizzas.** Using whole-wheat English muffins or tortillas, allow your children to make their own pizza with toppings like sliced turkey or chicken, tomato sauce, low-fat cheese, and chopped veggies of many colors (carrots, broccoli, eggplant, and so on).

- **Freeze some banana pops.** Slice a banana lengthwise and stick a popsicle stick in the middle. Offer your child a buffet of spreads like peanut butter, dark chocolate, or yogurt. Roll the banana in crushed cereal, nuts, or shredded coconut. Wrap and freeze for at least three hours.

- **Try frozen fruit cubes.** Freeze and puree three different color fruits separately, like strawberries, blueberries, and pineapple, and place into separate bowls. Allow your kids to scoop out colors into ice cube trays in any assortment they like. Cover and freeze for about three hours, pop out, and pop in your mouth!

- **Sneak in vitamins and minerals.** In smoothies or recipes for foods like muffins, sneak in pureed fruits and vegetables. Ask your children what type of smoothie they'd like and then add a dose of leafy greens or avocado. With muffins, replace half the oil in the recipe with applesauce or pureed pumpkin or add grated zucchini or carrots to the mix.

- **Getting creative.** There's a movement among mothers to break out of the brown bag and come up with creative Bento-like boxes for kids' school lunches. Instead of a PB&J sandwich and juice box, try putting a box together with lots of colors and foods in shapes such as rolled up turkey slices and melon balls or smaller sandwiches cut with cookie cutters into hearts and stars. Put faces on sandwiches and mini muffins using chocolate chips, cereal pieces, or whatever you have around the house. Not only can it be fun for your kid but it's also economical and eco-friendly!

Five steps to easing your spouse into it

I have a friend who essentially makes three different meals per night: a balanced meal for herself, a dish for their picky child eater, and another, heartier one for her husband. That takes a lot of time and energy, and if you're the one cooking, you may slack off on your own dish to ensure your spouse and child have their meals. With a bit of communication and clever thinking, you can get your spouse on the metabolism-boosting bandwagon and merge those meals into one.

✔ **Communicating:** Sit down and have a conversation with your spouse about the changes you want to make in your diet and why. Being open and honest about the foods you both enjoy and dislike, without getting offended about preparation, can help you put together meals and stock your kitchen with a balance of foods that can be healthy and nutritious.

✔ **Making small changes:** A complete overhaul of your diet can be unsustainable, and it can cause dissension among your family. Make sure you're involving your spouse in the process of revamping meals — and go slowly, one change at a time. For example, before trying new foods, try making healthy swaps in your family's favorite recipes.

✔ **Pointing out benefits:** What can be motivation for your spouse? Maybe they aren't concerned about weight but want to be able to keep up with your child's activity, or could reduce stress through more nutritious food choices. Pointing out how making changes can benefit both of you can keep you both motivated.

✔ **Showing support:** Don't focus on the negative aspects or berate your spouse for unhealthy habits. Recognize attempts to improve health, and the two of you can be amazing support for each other.

✔ **Being a good role model:** If you keep slacking off on your healthy habits, your spouse won't take you seriously. Practice what you preach. Seeing the positive results in you, your energy, mood, weight, and activity could encourage your spouse to do just the same.

For more ideas on incorporating healthy foods into your kids meals, check out the social media site Pinterest (`www.pinterest.com`). People all over the world are sharing ideas in the form of colorful pictures and links to quick and easy recipes.

Being active as a bunch

Do your typical family activities consist of watching television and arguing about bedtimes? Although having game night is a better, mind-stimulating use of your time, getting exercise as a group can kill two birds with one stone: getting a metabolism-boosting workout with the support from your loved ones.

Make activity a priority for at least one hour on the weekend and as much during the week as possible with your schedules. Don't let anything get in the way of that weekend time and don't let the weather stop you. Either bundle up or play an indoor game. Activity doesn't have to only mean sports like ice skating, basketball, swimming, biking, running, or walking. Although doing these as a group is a great, fun way to get your workout in. You can also:

- ✔ Have a dance party where each family member picks at least two songs.

- ✔ Try hula hooping and have a contest about who can keep theirs going the longest.

- ✔ Play games that kept people entertained before television and the Internet, such as hopscotch, jump rope, tug of war, and hide and seek.

- ✔ Go on family outings to the zoo or a park. Have a picnic and fly a kite. Take a trip to the mall or mini golf. Go camping to get out off the couch and out of the house.

Being active together helps improve your relationships and sets a good example for your children to grow up to be active people. If you face resistance, each week let a different family member choose the activity to compromise and keep everyone happy. In the end, all will have a sense of pride that they achieved something that day.

Also, any activity you're doing — whether you work your large muscle groups or not — helps burn additional calories. So even if you're not doing an intense workout at the gym, with your family you'll be helping your metabolic rate and instilling healthy habits in those around you.

Chapter 14

Smart Strategies for Eating On-The-Go

. . . .

In This Chapter

▶ Dining out and choosing the healthiest restaurant dishes

▶ Mastering the art of balanced eating when away from home

▶ Staying smart and social at parties while still boosting your metabolism

. . . .

*I*t can be relatively nice and easy staying on the metabolism-boosting bandwagon when you're at home, preparing all of your meals and snacks, knowing every ingredient that's going into your dish in the comfort of your kitchen. But take a step out the front door and you face temptation everywhere you go, from the lemonade stand run by your neighbor's kid, to the fare at a Mexican restaurant with friends, to traveling to your in-laws for the holidays (when stressful situations and decadent foods call you at every turn).

To keep your metabolism-boosting goals, should you stay at home or only eat foods you prep? No way! Are you going to be a hermit the rest of your life? Remember, it's not a good idea if it can't last long term. If you've ever been on a plan that offered pre-packaged or delivered meals, you may have been able to follow it for a short time. But they don't help when it comes to the difficult, real-life food situations you're bound to face in life. Mastering eating on-the-go is a sure sign that you're making lifestyle changes that can stick.

In this chapter, you'll see how to plan ahead for and handle times when you're faced with not-so-nutritious choices in restaurants, at the movies, at cocktail parties, or in front of an all-you-can-eat buffet. These don't need to be blowouts where you give up all hope of making healthy choices completely — nor do you need to go to extreme lengths to avoid the foods you love either. These situations can be anxiety provoking, and that's not a way to live either. You can give and take a little when on-the-go.

Dining Out Like a Metabolism Pro

When you eat in restaurants, you take in more calories than when you prepare foods at home (surprise, surprise!). It's not just fast-food joints that may contribute to packing on the pounds. Any sit-down restaurant can offer large portions laden with sauces and sides that add excess calories from saturated fat and sugar. And you may *really* be surprised when you learn the nutrition information of the foods you're eating when dining out.

Living in New York City, where there's only enough room for one person to walk into my kitchen, and where restaurants abound, I completely appreciate the need to dine out. No matter what size your kitchen is, you dine out to socialize, to celebrate, and to enjoy foods that you love. No one's telling you to give that up, especially not me. I'm here to help you stay on a diet that will still boost your metabolic rate and help you make the healthiest choices when in restaurants.

A closer look at calorie counts

Restaurants around the world list calorie counts next to their menu items to help consumers make more educated choices about their orders. The first wide-scale look at the impact of menu calorie counts, published in the *British Journal of Medicine*, found that one out of six people were actually affected by the information, and consumed about 100 calories less per meal. Although it may not seem like it, this is pretty significant. The information may not be perfect — and the calorie count alone doesn't tell the full story about the items — but it's still a way to gauge what you're taking in.

Another beneficial outcome from such labeling would be that restaurants could start offering more nutritious options and smaller portions — especially if such labels become mandatory, which is happening in some locales. Think about it, if a restaurant is required to post the calories, wouldn't that impact what the restaurant serves to please their health-conscious customers? In fact, when McDonald's took the initiative to post

their calories before a requirement was in place, they also added more healthful items to the menu.

Use the calorie count as a guide to make the better choice, but remember the following:

✔ The calories may appear as within a large range (based on optional components of the meal or accounting for a few items), so it can be difficult to pinpoint the exact number.

✔ Calorie counts may vary based on inconsistent serving sizes doled out by staff.

✔ There is more to a food than its caloric info that impacts your metabolic rate. Knowing the saturated fat, protein, sodium, fiber, and other nutrients is key for deciding whether or not a food is "worth" the calories. You can always ask the restaurant for additional information in-house or check online to see how the rest of the info matches up before making your choice.

Before leaving the house

Becoming a pro at dining out smart begins before you step out the door. If you're going to a restaurant with friends who order up a storm or pressure you into eating certain items, you need to go in prepared so you don't lose sight of your goals and lose mindfulness of what you're eating.

Here are some tips for setting yourself up for success before going out to a restaurant:

- **Studying the menu ahead of time:** Many if not most restaurant menus are online for you to look at and decide what can fit into your metabolism-boosting lifestyle. You may even find nutrition info, which is being listed more and more alongside menu items nationwide. If not, consider the cuisine and make a plan for what you'll order with some backups. For example, if it's Italian food, go for a grilled fish dish with a side of vegetables. If there's no fish, identify other lean proteins with healthy prep methods, like grilled chicken paillard. More on food choices by cuisine later in this section.

- **Having a snack:** If it's been more than three hours since your last meal, consider having a snack before leaving the house. Some fan favorites include a string cheese plus an apple, or a handful of nuts. If you snack smart, you won't go into the dinner ravenous, and you'll be more likely to keep your hands out of the bread basket.

- **Balancing the rest of your day:** You could be tempted to "save up calories" for a meal out. Although that seems like a good idea in theory, it usually doesn't pan out how you'd like it. If you restrict too much throughout the day, your energy levels will be lower, you may not be fueling your muscles properly if you're exercising, and you'll be even hungrier going into that dinner out, causing you to overeat. Instead, try to eat as balanced as possible during the rest of the day and don't dine out for other meals if you can help it. If you can't help it, follow the guidelines in this section for making the best choices you can when sitting down.

Strategizing restaurant menus and cuisines

Whether you're taking a look before you go online or you're opening up the menu as you sit down at the table, knowing the low-down on restaurant lingo can make all the difference when making healthy choices. Depending on where you're dining, you face unique challenges with the options available — from freebies on the table to accompanying cocktails to specific dishes.

When dealing with the freebies at restaurants such as bread or tortilla chips on the table, weigh your options:

✔ If you want bread or chips, take one serving from the main basket to your side plate. Make a concession elsewhere in the meal such as skipping an alcoholic drink, dessert, or starchy side (like pasta, potatoes, or additional bread with your meal).

✔ If you don't want it, ask the waiter to remove it from your table (of course, only if all your table companions feel the same way!).

✔ If you don't want the freebie but someone else at your table does, keep your mouth busy by drinking water and getting involved in conversation. Also, having a snack 2–3 hours prior to the meal will prevent you from going to the restaurant too hungry so that you can keep your hands out of the bread basket.

Prep methods can make or break the nutrient quality of the meal. See Table 14-1 for what to choose and what to lose when it comes to your favorite dishes.

Table 14-1	Restaurant Prep: Choose or Lose
Choose	*Lose*
Steamed	Sautéed
Broiled	Crispy
Stir-fry	Fried or pan-fried
Baked	Au gratin
Grilled	Scalloped
Poached	Creamed or buttered
Roasted	Stuffed or crusted

When in doubt, always ask your waiter about how a dish is prepared or how big the plate is. Often servers can be accommodating with menu substitutes and lighter methods if you simply speak up. Also, descriptive words may not tell the whole picture. Vegetables may be steamed, but they could also then be covered in butter sauce. Stir-fry is healthier than fried or pan-fried because less oil is used for a shorter period of time. However, often dishes that are stir-fried will have another sauce added on top of that such as soy sauce with cornstarch for thickening. See the upcoming section "Don't be saucy!" for more on how what your dish is topped with can sabotage your metabolism-boosting lifestyle.

Each cuisine presents its own hazards when navigating the options available to you. Table 14-2 should help you decide what to choose or lose, depending on the type of restaurant.

Table 14-2	Cuisine Choose or Lose	
Cuisine	*Choose*	*Lose*
Italian	Chicken paillard	Chicken or veal Parmigiana, Milanese
	Shrimp marinara	Shrimp scampi
	Whole-wheat pasta primavera	White pasta Bolognese
	House salad, oil and vinegar	Tomato and mozzarella
	Steamed spinach	Zucchini fritti
Mexican	Seafood ceviche	Nachos
	Chicken fajitas (tortillas used sparingly)	Steak burrito or tacos
	Side of black beans	Fried plantains
	Guacamole (2 tablespoons)	Jalapeno poppers
	Tequila with club soda, lime	Frozen margarita
Chinese	Steamed chicken or shrimp or tofu with veggies	General Tso's chicken
	Moo goo gai pan (stir-fry)	Beef with broccoli
	Brown rice	White rice or noodles
	Steamed dim sum	Egg roll
	Fresh pineapple	Green tea ice cream
Indian	Chicken tikka or tandoori	Chicken korma or tikki masala
	Roti (whole wheat)	Stuffed naan
	Lentil soup	Samosa
Steakhouse	Petite filet mignon	Rib eye or prime rib
	Shrimp cocktail	Fried calamari or crab cake
	Grilled tuna steak	Filet of sole Francese
	Plain baked potato	Crispy onions
	Grilled asparagus	Creamed spinach

Restaurant menus can be deceiving. Just because a dish sounds like the healthier option doesn't always make it the best choice when out to eat. Don't make these common restaurant mistakes:

✔ **Olive oil with bread:** Although oil is a healthier alternative to butter, you can still soak up 120 calories *per tablespoon* when dipping your bread into olive oil. Either dip lightly or skip altogether.

✔ **Small plates or tapas:** Portion control heaven, right? Not always. When out to eat at tapas, it's often hard to remember how much you've eaten when multiple plates keep coming out of the kitchen and you take bites off every one. On top of that, if the items are fried or sautéed, you may be getting more than you bargained for. When choosing small plates with a table, put in a request for ceviches, grilled meats, and veggies.

✔ **Salads:** Although you may be getting a dose of vegetables with a salad, you may also be getting the caloric equivalent of a hamburger. At Applebee's, for example, the Grilled Shrimp and Spinach Salad clocks in at over 1,000 calories — which is about the equivalent of their Steak and Riblets Combo. Items to watch for and exclude from salads include creamy dressings, croutons, cheese, bacon, flash fried or breaded protein sources, and the list goes on. Ask what's in your salad, make swaps, and ask for all dressings on the side.

✔ **Vegetarian and vegan:** Eggplant Parmigiana, cheese ravioli, vegetable burritos, and fried tofu are just a few examples of ways restaurants infuse saturated fat and sodium into seemingly innocent meatless dishes. Sometimes meat or fish can be a better option depending on the preparation method and what else is on the dish.

Don't be saucy!

If there's one piece of advice you should take from me when dining out, make it this:

Get sauces served on the side! Sauces are often a hidden (or not so hidden) source of calories, carbohydrates, fat, and sodium.

Although sauces, dressings, and condiments do add flavor to a dish, requesting for them to be served on the side or making swaps can help you control the amount that goes in to help keep tabs on outlandish calorie counts.

Here are some saucy tips:

✔ Ask for salad dressing on the side or no-mayo on your sandwich bun to save at least 200 calories and 20 grams of fat.

✔ Substitute grilled chicken for BBQ chicken and save about 100 calories, 400 milligrams of sodium, and 30 grams of carbohydrate.

✔ Request your sweet and sour Chinese dish be steamed with sauce served on the side and save about 400 calories, 700 milligrams of sodium, and 60 grams of carbohydrate.

✔ Skip cheese sauce on a broccoli side dish and save 200 calories, 16 grams of fat, and 1,000 milligrams of sodium.

✔ Request your steak be cooked without seasoned butter sauce and save 400 calories, 50 grams of fat (30 grams saturated fat), and 500 milligrams of sodium.

✔ Choose marinara sauce instead of Alfredo sauce and save at least 140 calories and 15 grams of fat.

✔ Skip gravy on mashed potatoes and save about 150 calories and up to 1,200 milligrams of sodium.

Eating right through summer nights

The summer season presents its own challenges when it comes to sticking to healthy habits on-the-go. As the weather turns warmer, your calendar gets filled up with more social events that are full of food challenges, such as barbecues, ballgames, and going to the movies to escape the heat. Don't let your lazy summer translate into a lazy metabolism. You can still be mindful of making better choices, even with more indulgent foods. Steer clear of jumbo, sugary beverages and pay close attention to portions to make the best choices you can at these events on your calendar:

✔ **Block party barbecue:** Worst choices: Fried chicken, spareribs, sausage, potato salad, chips, lemonade. Best choices: Grilled chicken, sirloin, fish, corn on the cob, collard greens, watermelon.

✔ **Take me out to the ballgame:** Worst choices: Corn dogs, nachos, cotton candy, soft pretzels. Best choices: Peanuts, small hot dog, small soft serve ice cream cone.

✔ **Going to the Movies:** Worst choices: Soda, buttered popcorn, large boxes of candy. Best choices: Small unbuttered popcorn, small box of candy (split with a friend).

Although olive oil is a heart-healthy source of fats, vegetables like eggplant and mushrooms can soak up much of what's in the pan and add a lot of calories to otherwise low-calorie vegetables. Request that your dish be prepared steamed and ask for olive oil on the side to add yourself or "light on oil" to keep flavor without too much fat.

Making a meal out of appetizers and sides

The way a dish is prepared isn't the only reason restaurant dishes average between 1,000–1,500 calories per plate! Because of ever-expanding portion sizes of meals for one, your entree alone can take up a large proportion of an entire day's worth of calories — not to mention what else you order up like drinks, appetizers, and sides. To eyeball what a serving size and portion should look like, see Chapter 6.

Pair appetizers and sides to create your meal instead of an entrée to control the amount you're given in restaurants (and ultimately the amount you eat) while still giving you a variety, so you don't feel deprived. Unless they're served family style, appetizers and sides can offer up instant portion control and a dose of metabolism-boosting foods.

- Pair lean proteins with fiber from whole grains, fruits, or vegetables so that you're satisfied. Here are some examples:
  - Appetizer of grilled/raw seafood plus a side of whole-wheat pasta
  - Appetizer of spinach salad plus lentil soup appetizer
  - Side of roasted vegetables plus a side of hummus plus whole-wheat pita
  - Appetizer of grilled chicken kebab skewer plus a side fruit salad
  - Appetizer of edamame plus an appetizer of sashimi salad

- Ask your waiter about approximate sizes of the plates so you can determine whether pairing an appetizer and side is not enough food or too much.

- Don't ignore prep methods. Just because the plate is smaller doesn't mean it doesn't pack a calorie punch from fried, sautéed dishes, with butter, cream sauce, or cheeses.

If none of the side dishes fit into your metabolism-boosting meal plan, cut the calorie count of your meal and:

- **Go halvsies.** Split an entrée with a friend.

- **Bring a doggy bag.** Pack up half your dish even before you start eating.

✔ **Downsize the dish.** Some restaurants are jumping on the bandwagon of offering smaller portions at a reduced price. There's no harm in asking!

✔ **Revoke your membership in the clean plate club.** If you're the type who must finish their plate, eat slowly so that you can pay attention to your physical hunger cues (if you're not sure how, see Chapter 6). The more you practice, the easier it'll get to leave food on your plate and stop when you're satisfied instead of becoming uncomfortably full. Or you can always practice the doggy bag tip mentioned earlier.

All-you-can eat buffets are the most difficult place to control your portions and calorie counts due to a plethora of options and no limit on servings. If you have a choice of where to dine, avoid these places. If you don't have a choice, learn how to make the best choices when faced with a spread at a party, later in this chapter.

Traveling Like a Pro

If you regularly find yourself in airports, rest stops, and faced with vending machine snack options, you already know that when traveling, you don't come across the most metabolism-friendly places. Whether you're traveling for work or leisure, making flights and sticking to itineraries is hectic enough, so you may let all your healthy habits go out the window. Instead, pack the knowledge from this section in your suitcase so that you can get to your destination with your metabolism intact.

Packing snacks

Clothes and toiletries packed. Check. Car full of gas, plane or train ticket, photo ID, itinerary set. Check, check, and check. Healthy snacks packed? If this isn't on your standard list of travel needs, it should be — just like you need a book or magazine to read on the train.

The word *snack* gets a bad rap. Many automatically think of vending machine potato chips, candy, or chocolate and decide that cutting out snacking between meals would be an effective way to lose weight. Not so! Snacks are important because going too many hours between meals and getting too hungry can impair your judgment when on-the-go.

When traveling, you never know if you'll hit traffic or a flight delay, prolonging the time before you find your next metabolism-boosting meal. Having a snack on hand helps keep your energy high and metabolism strong throughout a hectic traveling day or when you're in a new place.

Pack non-perishable snacks that you can throw in your carry-on bag or suitcase without worry:

- ✔ Low-fat granola, protein, or cereal bars

- ✔ Dried fruits like apricots, mango, or dates

- ✔ Unsalted nuts like pistachios, walnuts, almonds, or soy nuts

- ✔ Seeds like pumpkin or sunflower seeds

- ✔ Nut butters like almond or peanut butter, which also come in individual serving packs

- ✔ 100-calorie dark chocolate bars (as long as it's not too hot out)

- ✔ Baked chips like whole-wheat pita chips, soy chips, or apple or vegetable chips

- ✔ Baked, high-fiber crackers

- ✔ Vacuum-packed pouches of albacore light tuna, chicken, or salmon

If you're taking a road trip or packing snacks for a day at the beach, you'll have more room and flexibility with what you can bring along. Why not bring a cooler with ice packs to keep food cold and fresh and reduce your risk of food-borne illness? Plan ahead so that foods available at gas station rest stops or beach snack bars aren't your only options:

- ✔ Whole-grain bread sandwiches with nut butter, hummus, or lean meats like chicken and turkey

- ✔ Fresh cut-up fruit and vegetables

- ✔ Low-fat string cheese, soy cheese, or spreadable cheeses to put on high-fiber crackers

- ✔ Low-fat yogurt, milk, or soy milk boxes

- ✔ Plenty of water in aluminum water bottles to stay hydrated

Eating smart at airports and rest stops

Of course, you can't always plan ahead. And sometimes you're just stuck out of your element and need to make the best choices you can when waiting for your flight or during a road trip. Unfortunately, most of the options available don't pack a nutritional punch and instead will fill you up with those metabolism-busters like saturated fat, sugar, and sodium, leaving you feeling sluggish and sleepy (far from ideal if you're driving!).

Many airports are jumping on a healthy-option bandwagon, and you can bypass fast-food joints for cafes that offer fresh fruits, oatmeal, yogurts, sandwiches, and salads. However, fast-food chains are still more prevalent in airports and on the road.

Here are your best bets in those situations:

✔ At a coffee chain, choose a skim latte for a pick-me-up with a dose of protein and calcium. Skip the added sugar flavors or whipped cream.

✔ At a sandwich chain, make your own sandwich with whole-grain bread, lean meats, and veggies. Skip the cheese, mayo, and excess sauces.

✔ At a pastry chain, seek out a whole-grain bagel with light cream cheese or an egg sandwich. Skip sugary, frosting-covered donuts as well as the airport staple: cinnamon buns.

✔ At a pizza chain, request thin crust pizza with a vegetable topping — if possible, with whole-wheat crust and little cheese. Add a side salad to help fill you up and skip stuffed-crust or meat-laden pies.

✔ On a flight, just because the stewardess hands you a salty snack like nuts doesn't mean you have to eat it if you're not hungry. Skip sodas and alcohol in flight as well and opt for water or seltzer instead because you're more prone to get dehydrated on board (due to lack of moisture in the air in the cabin). This will help keep your energy high and prevent you from indulging to help offset fatigue later on.

Hydrating on vacation

Throughout my childhood, my family was keen getting enough water, especially if we were on the beach on vacation. I remember my brother always said, "Hydration is key," although I never really understood what he meant. Now I know it's because our bodies are composed of up to 60 percent water, and our brains up to 70 percent. Not re-filling the water lost through excretion or sweat can cause fatigue and nausea.

What my family probably wasn't alluding to is the fact that water helps boost your metabolism:

✔ Each of your cells requires water for basic functioning, such as converting food into energy and transporting nutrients to other cells. Without water, cells aren't working the best they can — which is the root of your metabolic rate.

> ✔ Drink cold water, and your body temperature may rise to counteract the cold, resulting in a slightly increased calorie burn.
>
> ✔ Being dehydrated may manifest in feelings of hunger, causing you to seek out food or an ice cream treat from the beach snack bar to cool down.

The Institute of Medicine (IOM) recommendations adequate fluid intake of 91 ounces for women and 125 ounces for men per day. Remember that you do take in fluids from food and other beverages besides water, so in this case, you'd be in the clear drinking about eight to twelve 8-ounce cups of water every day.

On vacation or during a busy travel schedule, you can easily forget to drink enough water. And you may need even more in warmer temperatures or when you're very active and sweating. Make it a priority by carrying a bottle with you everywhere you go or keeping a glass next to your chair on the beach. Remember, hydration is key!

Navigating a Party

From hors d'oeuvres to all-you-can-eat buffets to desserts and cocktails, thinking about all of the temptations presented at a party can be anxiety provoking. Especially around the wedding and holiday seasons, but year-round for birthdays and special occasions, many of my clients tell me it's impossible to make changes to their diet because of unlimited food and drink at parties.

Yes, food and drinks are usually present, but the party is about so much more than that. Instead of hyper-focusing on how you're going to avoid temptation, think about the people you'll see there, get involved in conversation with old friends and new people, because social events are, after all, about interacting with others.

In this section, you'll find out how to feel like you're a part of the party, satisfied from the food and drinks you're consuming and enjoying yourself, without overdoing it on calories.

Being appetizer and buffet savvy

A party with tasty-looking appetizers or buffet can be your worst nightmare, but don't let it get the best of you.

Here's how you can keep your calories in check around such feasts:

- ✔ **Ask ahead about the food that'll be offered at any affair.** That way you'll know if just hors d'oeuvres are being served or foods that aren't in line with your metabolism-boosting lifestyle, to have a more substantial snack or light meal even before you head out.

- ✔ **Don't save up your calories to eat at a buffet.** If you go too many hours without eating before the party and during cocktail hour you only munch on carrot sticks, you're going to be ravenous and feel your resolve weaken when faced with tables and tables of indulgent food. Have a snack before the party and choose only one of your high-fat, calorie favorite hors d'oeuvres (mine is pigs in a blanket) before heading into the main event. Otherwise, stick to the raw bar, crudité (light on the dips), and grilled chicken skewers you typically find at cocktail hour.

- ✔ **Don't be a professional sampler.** Typically, the more variety you have either during the cocktail hours or at a buffet, the more you'll eat over-all. Just as you choose one favorite in the cocktail hour, choose only one serving of a food that's outside the healthy box at the buffet. Scope out what's available before picking your favorite and opt for an item you don't typically eat. By doing a lap before you commit to food choices, you'll also have an educated view of what the best options are instead of grabbing whatever's for the taking.

- ✔ **Remember that sauce isn't calorie free.** When you scoop a dish onto your plate, skimp on the amount of sauce or dressing you pick up in the spoon. Also, try to limit picking foods from the bottom of the pan, which have soaked up more of the oil or sauce used during preparation.

- ✔ **Make a plate and step away from the buffet.** When making a dinner plate for yourself, consider the plate method. Make half your plate vegetables and fruit, one quarter of it starch like potato, rice, or pasta, and one quarter lean protein like chicken, fish, or beans. Use a smaller plate if available so you pile on less. Then walk away and try to park yourself at a table far away from the buffet so you're less tempted to go back for more.

- ✔ **Eat with your stomach.** Often, your eyes may be bigger than your stomach, and the signs that you're full can get muted by alcohol or too much stimulation from people. Or you've just served too much on your plate to begin with. Pay attention to whether you're really hungry or full before getting up for seconds. If you do feel hungry for seconds, don't choose the high-fat, high-calorie food you vowed to only have one serving of. Instead, go for salads and vegetables, broth-based soups, or a small piece of grilled fish to help fill you up the metabolism-boosting way: lots of volume, low on calories.

✔ **Don't forget about water.** Keep drinking water throughout the meal so you stay hydrated, don't confuse thirst with hunger, and fill up a bit faster to help prevent overeating.

✔ **Mind your cocktails.** It's a party, go ahead and have a drink or two. Having a drink in your hand during a cocktail party can actually be great — your hands are less available to grab an appetizer off every plate that passes. That drink doesn't always have to be alcoholic, but if it is, follow these guidelines:

  • Choose wine, beer, or liquor on the rocks or with a no-calorie mixer, like seltzer or club soda, or a splash of juice.

  • Skip any frozen or mixed cocktails with juice or soda which are packed with calories from sugar.

  • Don't drink on an empty stomach and alternate an alcoholic drink with a glass of water so that you don't get too tipsy, which can adversely impact your food decisions.

Indulging your sweet tooth

If you want to have dessert, there's no shame in that at a party — but there are ways to minimize the blow to your metabolism.

✔ **Stick to single servings.** Take one small cookie or brownie from a dessert buffet table instead of bringing a variety plate back to your table. Then have a cup of tea or decaf coffee to help keep your hands busy and prevent you from going back for more.

✔ **Serve yourself a sliver.** Research shows that people dish out more when serving others than they do when grabbing a portion for themselves. Therefore, slice your own sliver of pie or cake. If the hostess hands you a large piece, split it with someone at your table.

✔ **Choose fruit as a filler.** If you have a sliver of cake or a cookie and still don't feel satisfied, instead of getting a second serving of that, fill your plate with fiber-rich fruit. Or only choose fruit in the first place to help satisfy your sweet tooth without breaking the calorie bank.

Indulging in a dessert every once in awhile is important so you don't go overboard with portions at parties. When you tell yourself it's okay to have dessert, you're less likely to idealize and crave it. Chapter 4 talks about breaking out of black-and-white thinking so that you can ditch the deprivation mentality, achieve a balance, and still lose weight.

Asserting your healthy choices

You may feel like you're not strong enough to stick to your convictions and make healthy choices at a party. Maybe in the past you've gone to events with the best intentions but returned home feeling overstuffed and defeated.

In addition to planning a strategy for what you'll eat and drink ahead of time, being assertive with your healthy choices can make them a reality:

- ✔ **Just say no.** You don't have to explain to your aunt why you're not trying the chocolate cake she made special for the holiday party or go back and forth with your friend about why you don't want a second glass of wine. Just say "No, thank you," and change the topic of conversation. If someone keeps insisting, say that you'd rather not and you'd appreciate it if they respected your decision.

- ✔ **Take one bite.** You may be handed a plate of dessert or find yourself in a work setting where you don't want to eat or go into detail about your healthy lifestyle or the food choices you make. Take one bite and get distracted by the company around you. Make it about the conversation, not about the food. You shouldn't feel obligated to finish your plate just to be polite.

- ✔ **You're #1.** Your health and well-being must be your priority. Don't worry about how others will feel bad or be offended if you don't eat their home-prepared food. They'll get over it. If you're in a position where you need to explain your actions, say that eating nutritiously makes you feel good, gives you energy, and your goal is to have a healthy and happy life. Who could argue with that? Certainly not someone who has your best intentions at heart. Put up a fight for making the choices you need to in the name of your metabolism-boosting lifestyle — no matter where you are.

Part V
The Part of Tens

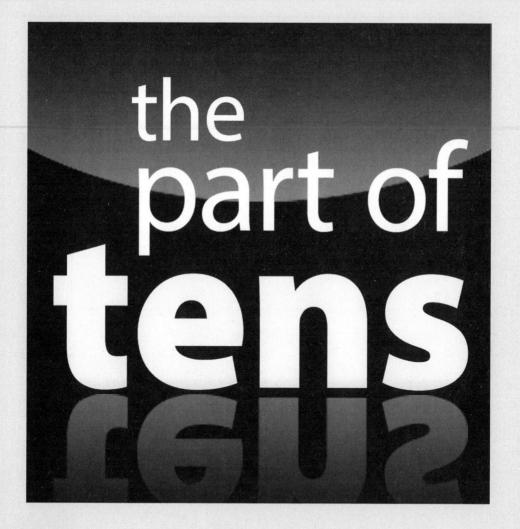

Enjoy an additional metabolism-boosting Part of Tens chapter online at www.dummies.com/extras/boostingyourmetabolism.

In this part . . .

- ✔ Find out how to tell whether you're really boosting your metabolism with ten sure signs.

- ✔ Keep your stomach's growls at bay with ten tips on fighting cravings.

- ✔ Don't believe everything you hear or read — dispelling ten metabolism myths.

Chapter 15

Ten Sure Signs You're Boosting Your Metabolism

· ·

In This Chapter

▶ Reaping the health benefits of an improved metabolism

▶ Measuring your progress as you change your lifestyle

· ·

*A*s you improve your diet to boost your metabolism, you experience changes in your body and your mind. Seeing these positive changes helps keep you motivated to continue down a healthy path.

Remember, this is a marathon, not a sprint. Take rest stops along the way to track how far you've really come.

Just because you don't see immediate weight loss, that's not a reason to bow out of the race and give up. Many factors are in play when it comes to your metabolism, and weight is definitely not the only indicator of health. Take a look at all these signs and numbers, instead of just your weight, to measure your progress and gauge your success in improving your metabolic rate.

Weight Loss

According to the World Health Organization, about 1.6 billion people in the world are overweight or obese (see Chapter 2 for a definition of these terms), and at least 2.5 million deaths are attributed to obesity-related conditions every year. Being overweight or obese also often carries a hefty price tag in medical bills and associated conditions such as diabetes, heart disease, high blood pressure, and metabolic syndrome. Losing weight has numerous health benefits and can improve mobility, energy levels, and confidence to take on whatever life has in store for you.

By consuming nutrient-dense foods such as fresh fruits and vegetables, lean meats and fish, low-fat dairy, and heart-healthy fats like nuts and seeds, you stoke your metabolism and reduce your waistline. Choosing a balance of those nutrients for every meal and snack, plus not going too many hours between eating, helps keep your metabolism moving as effectively as possible. You're burning more calories while taking in higher-quality nutrients, resulting in a declining number on the scale.

Building lean muscle mass through regular exercise can help you burn even more calories at rest. Because muscle weighs more than fat, in the beginning of an exercise regimen you might not see much weight change. But keep in mind that muscle tissue will make up for it in the long run.

Better Energy

A sluggish metabolism means a sluggish you. If you've ever noticed a correlation between what you eat or the exercise you do and the amount of energy you have, then you've got a clue what I'm talking about. If you haven't yet made any changes to your eating or activity levels, you're in for a treat. Feeding the body the nutrients it needs — really fueling it properly — helps charge you up with the energy you need to excel throughout the day.

On the metabolism plan, you no longer skip meals, focus on a balance of nutrients, drink plenty of water, and move your body in one way or another every day. When your meals consist of plenty of lean protein and complex carbohydrates, you feel fuller longer which keeps that energy level elevated.

Boosting your metabolism has numerous positive effects on your productivity and mood. You'll be making the most of what life has to offer for you, and many of my clients say the boost in energy is the best daily reminder that they've improved their metabolic rate.

Here are just some of the benefits of boosting your energy:

- ✔ Easier time waking up in the morning.
- ✔ No more mid-morning or mid-afternoon crash-and-burns.
- ✔ Making time for exercise doesn't seem like such a chore.
- ✔ Able to slowly improve the quality and quantity of your activity.

Improved Cholesterol Levels

Although high cholesterol levels on their own don't cause symptoms, they do increase your risk for a cardiac event and heart disease. Your body does require cholesterol to create hormones and to digest and absorb certain nutrients. But when the levels get out of whack, it can cause build-up of plaque in your arteries, often leading to heart attack or stroke. Your vulnerability depends on your age, sex, genetics, weight, lifestyle, and past medical history.

If you're over 20, you should get your lipoprotein profile checked once every 5 years. These are the levels you want to see:

- **LDL ("bad") cholesterol:** Less than 100
- **HDL ("good") cholesterol:** Higher than 60
- **Triglycerides (circulating fat in your blood):** Less than 150

As you minimize foods that are high in saturated and trans fats and refined sugar, you can expect your LDL and triglycerides to decrease. Including more of the "goods" — like omega-3 fatty acids, fiber, plant stanols and sterols, and plenty of activity — will help balance out wonky cholesterol levels. Many of the lifestyle changes you make when improving your metabolism will help your lipoprotein profile. In any case, this gives you more numbers to track besides weight.

Better Digestion

When your metabolism is slow, it typically also means that your digestion isn't up to snuff or you aren't eating the right stuff. When your body isn't digesting foods properly, you might experience constipation, bloating, reflux, and general discomfort along your gastrointestinal tract. Consuming unrefined foods like whole grains, fruits, and veggies provides more fiber, which keeps your digestive system moving well. Minimizing refined, processed foods, alcohol, and caffeine takes away substances that can interfere with digestion. Getting enough good ol' H_2O helps keep your gut happy. If you've ever suffered from gastrointestinal stress, you know how much it can affect your daily life, and how much better you feel when it's resolved.

Your stomach and brain are very in tune with each other. When you feel anxious or stressed, it can either diminish your appetite or cause you to overeat. Just one more reason to learn how to relax and take care of your health physically and mentally. Getting enough sleep and regular activity are also integral parts of this healthy gut equation. See Chapter 4 for more.

Reduced Stress

You might have heard of *stress eating*, which usually relates to overeating when under stress. But did you know that not eating enough or the right types of foods can actually *lead* to stress? Following any type of diet in which you aren't satisfying your body's needs leaves it feeling deprived. When your brain isn't getting the fuel it needs to tell the muscles what to do, all goes awry. Consider these questions:

- ✔ Have you cut out a nutrient group like carbs, fat, or protein?
- ✔ Do you constantly think about food and/or your weight?
- ✔ Do you feel anxious when dining out?
- ✔ Do you avoid social situations where you can't control the food that's served?

If you answer yes to any of those questions, your diet may be making you stressed out. Balance is key for success; don't think of food in terms of "black and white." Being comfortable with having both a balance of protein, carbs, and fat — and a balance between nutritious and "fun" foods — will keep you satisfied on a physical and mental level.

Improved Circulation

Are you always cold? That can be a sign of a slow metabolism. A lifetime of fatty foods causes plaque build-up in your arteries, which constricts your veins. Smoking cigarettes and lack of exercise can also constrict the flow of molecules, resulting in feeling cold in your extremities, cramping, and numbness. Poor circulation is also a symptom of hypothyroidism, a disorder of metabolism.

Certain foods can help with improved circulation. Antioxidants from fruits and vegetables spanning all colors of the rainbow improve the health of your blood vessels and, therefore, circulation. Consuming a serving of lean protein at each meal provides you with amino acids, which assist in transporting molecules through your body. Kicking that cigarette habit and making time for movement while you're at it can help improve blood flow and circulation.

More Strength

Building and maintaining lean muscle mass helps boost your metabolic rate. With strength training, you'll expend additional calories during the workout, following the workout (increased caloric burn for 24–48 hours), and ultimately burn more calories at rest if you keep the lean muscle mass. Think beyond weights. Combine different activities and keep your muscles guessing. See Chapter 11 for more info on the best exercises to boost your metabolic rate.

Diet and exercise go hand in hand. Lean protein helps create and strengthen muscles that are active. Foods like chicken, turkey, fish, lean beef, nuts, seeds, beans, and whole grains can help you meet your muscle needs. Fueling up with complex carbohydrates helps those muscles recover and maximize endurance for any activity you do.

By engaging in varieties of resistance, cardio, and isometric exercises, you can enjoy benefits such as improved posture, mobility, better sleep, and more self-confidence.

Lowered Blood Pressure

If your blood pressure is regularly elevated because of your weight, stress, or other genetic or lifestyle factors, and you've been put on medication to help control it, the steps you take to improve your metabolism will help lower your blood pressure and can reduce your need for medication. These steps include the following:

✔ Ditching the salt shaker and processed foods to reduce the sodium in your diet

✔ Getting more potassium from fruits and veggies

✔ Including foods like cayenne pepper and green tea in your diet

Boosted Immune System

Want to boost your immune system? Make sure that you:

✔ Fuel up with good nutrition

✔ Get moving with activity

✔ Chill out to reduce stress

It's no coincidence that those are the three main aspects you focus on to boost your metabolism. Instead of just improving on one or the other, you reap the benefits of all three for your immune system, to keep you strong and help prevent disease.

Antioxidants are those power nutrients found in all types of fruits, veggies, whole grains, nuts, and seeds that work to eliminate free radicals caused by environmental factors like cigarette smoking and pollution. Free radicals can cause damage to your DNA, and contribute to artery plaque and diseases like cancer, heart disease, and even the common cold and flu. Eating from the rainbow — a variety of produce — can help you get more types of these antioxidants to fight those free radicals.

Walk for 30 minutes at least 5 days per week. Or if you can't do it all at once, break it up into ten-minute intervals, three times per day. Research shows this bolsters the antibody response integral to your immune system. It's not clear whether it's a direct benefit or if walking improves mental function that in turn boosts immunity. But either way, walking, and any activity, can also reduce stress and improve your circulation, which also helps all systems of your body work efficiently.

Better Blood Sugar Control

Whether or not you have diabetes or are at risk of developing it, everyone can benefit from better blood sugar control. Ups and downs of blood sugar can lead to food cravings, impaired judgment when it comes to your food choices, fatigue, and just a plain old cranky mood. With the foundation of a metabolism meal plan ensuring that you eat every 4–5 hours with plenty of fiber and without refined sugars, spikes in your blood sugar will be better in control. This means a waterfall effect of nutritious food choices, more energy to get the activity you need, and feeling your best inside and out.

Chapter 16

Ten Tips to Fight Cravings

In This Chapter

▶ Preventing cravings with your metabolism-boosting lifestyle

▶ Understanding when and how you should give in to cravings

*F*ood cravings can come on fast and hit you hard. One minute you're sitting on your couch watching TV, and the next minute you're foraging through your kitchen cabinets looking for the box of cookies you pushed towards the back to hide them.

Not all food cravings come from a physical need to eat. They also come from the pleasure derived from eating, which is often used as a means to try to deal with negative emotions.

Your stomach and brain are strongly connected. Hormones are released when your stomach is empty or full to tell your brain you should eat or stop eating. But food cravings go beyond basic hunger mechanisms. Because high-fat and sugary foods release substances that give your brain a sense of euphoria, you're also seeking that feeling. That's why a line is often drawn between food cravings and addiction; addiction to food may be not as strong as drugs, but it uses the same pathway nonetheless. Yet, as this chapter makes clear, restricting those foods isn't the answer.

So what is the answer? How you eat isn't totally out of your control if you're prone to cravings. Many of the tips from the metabolism-boosting diet discussed in this book are engineered to minimize food cravings. Winning the fight over food cravings is about both the physical and the psychological. These ten tips address both sides of the equation to encourage you to listen to your body and develop a healthier relationship with food.

Ditch the "Diet" Mentality

When you restrict what you eat too severely, it backfires in the long run. A study published in *Appetite* out of Hertfordshire University found that women who tried to suppress their cravings for chocolate ate 50 percent *more* than those who were encouraged to talk about and indulge their craving. A ton of research shows that when you try to push a thought out of your mind, you end up thinking about it even more, making the desire stronger and stronger. Another study found that *restrained* eaters — those who eliminate a food group or severely restrict their calories — were more likely to indulge and overeat the restricted food when given the opportunity.

Eating less than 1,200 calories a day can leave you feeling deprived, and over a prolonged period of time it can slow your metabolic rate. (See Chapter 3 to find out how many calories your body needs for healthy, sustainable weight loss, gain, or maintenance, depending on your goals.)

Similarly, going more than five hours between meals can cause a drop in your blood sugar level, which brings cravings on with a vengeance. This leaves you vulnerable to making unhealthy choices and hitting up the first drive-thru you see.

Snack is not a bad word. A snack is necessary when you have a long stretch between meals.

Break Your Habits

Do you always have a soda with your lunch or a box of chocolate candy whenever you go to the movies? When you start eating foods out of habit, you'll crave that food when you're in each situation, and probably not even think twice about it. You can retrain your brain to make healthier choices:

- ✔ Stop and think before you eat or drink. Ask yourself if you're truly hungry and if you really need or want the food.

- ✔ Plan ahead. Come up with an alternative to your habit, such as choosing seltzer water with lunch or splitting a small popcorn, no butter, with your friend at the movies.

- ✔ To reduce your larger than normal portions at home, switch to smaller serving plates or portion out a serving instead of eating out of the bulk container.

- ✔ If you typically indulge in cookies, cakes, and other goodies brought in by your coworkers, ask yourself, *would I pay for this?* If not, skip it and keep more nutritious options in your desk drawer.

Distract Yourself

Cravings come in waves, meaning they don't last forever. They build up, reach a peak, and then subside. If you ride it out during the peak by distracting yourself, it's possible that enough time will pass until the craving eases up. Keep a list of items you can do to distract yourself on your refrigerator or somewhere easily accessible so you can do a little less thinking when your mind is consumed by the thought of a food. Include on your list activities that help you relax, like taking a bath. Or keep your mind entertained with a book. Or surf the Internet so you can also surf past the craving wave.

Even if you end up indulging, if you manage to put five more minutes between craving the food and actually eating it, that's a win. Next time, you'll wait 30 minutes, the next time an hour … eventually, you'll develop the strength not to give in to a craving if you're not really hungry.

Get Your ZZZs

Anything less than seven hours of sleep per night, and your hormones that signal appetite can get out of whack, making you more likely to overeat. A study out of University of Chicago found that just two nights of getting four hours of sleep can have this effect and that cravings for sweet, salty, and starchy foods increased as a result. When you're running on no sleep, you might find yourself more vulnerable for these cravings and give in with hope that the food will help "wake you up."

A good night's sleep is just as important as a day of nutritious food and physical activity. See my free online article "Taking Care to Change Your Lifestyle" at www.dummies.com/extras/boostingyourmetabolism/ for details on why sleep affects your appetite and how to get your seven hours minimum.

When you just can't get enough sleep, take five minutes in the morning to plan meals and snacks. Ideally, these meals will contain a balance of lean protein, high fiber, and heart-healthy carbohydrates to help give you the nutrients you need to get through the day.

Stay Hydrated

If you think you're experiencing a food craving, but it's not time for your meal or snack, drink a glass of water — you might actually be thirsty. When you're dehydrated, you often feel fatigued because your body is comprised of about 60 percent water. That water needs replenishing to keep you energized and your digestive systems moving. Before you reach for food, think about whether you've had enough water that day, especially if you're in a warm climate or have been more active than usual.

If it's tough for you to get enough water because of the boring taste, add a few berries, lemon juice, or cucumber slices to your glass for a sweet, tart, or refreshing flavor. Also, always keep a glass of water within arm's reach: an aluminum water bottle on-the-go, on your nightstand to remind you to drink first thing in the morning, or a pitcher on your desk at work. You can also set an alert on your cell phone to remind you to drink your water and when in doubt about how much to gulp, let thirst be your guide.

Savor the Heat

The spicy component of chili peppers, capsaicin, has been shown to increase energy expenditure post-meal and suppress your appetite. Adding chili peppers in your diet can not only increase your metabolic rate but also enhance the flavor of nutritious foods — making you more likely to eat them. Also, if you're not used to the heat, it can help you slow down when eating, which in turn can help you recognize physical signs of fullness sooner so that you eat less overall.

If you're craving something decadent, a spicy food — maybe some hot sauce drizzled on hummus for your veggie dip or chopped up chili peppers mixed in with a broth-based soup — could do the trick for fewer calories. Try adding chili pepper to anything from eggs to meat and fish to fruit salad.

Move It!

Walking away from the "trouble" spot physically removes you from the food craving situation. However, any kind of exercise you do can also activate those pleasure receptors in your brain to release endorphins that make you happy and reduce stress. Therefore, not only is exercise essential to keeping your metabolism working the best it can, it also can reduce food cravings throughout the day. Here are a few tips:

✔ **Get started slowly and make it more enjoyable.** If you're forcing yourself to do intense workouts at the gym, which you hate, it's not going to last. Try a group exercise class on your level or invest in a workout DVD that looks interesting to you.

> ✔ **Think about the best, most realistic time of day for you to make time for activity.** For example, maybe you can create a habit of going for a walk every night after dinner.

> ✔ **Buddy up for accountability and to create healthy habits with your family and friends.** You're much more likely to wake up early for that exercise class if you know a friend will be there waiting for you.

See Chapter 11 for more activity ideas suitable for all skill levels.

Picture Your Progress

Sometimes when the craving strikes, just picturing your goals — how you want to look or feel, or the results you want when you visit the doctor's office — can be a powerful way to prevent you from indulging. One reason this works is that it helps you increase awareness about what you're doing if it's consistent with what you're trying to achieve. When you're craving something sweet, and you picture a lower number for your weight on the doctor's scale, you might think twice about reaching for that jelly donut.

Thinking back on how far you've come is also helpful. Track your progress by keeping a food, activity, and weight journal. When you're having difficulty sticking to healthy habits, look at this record of what's worked and what hasn't worked for you in the past so you can stay motivated for the future.

Watch Processed Sugars

If there's one type of food you need to monitor and minimize in your diet to reduce cravings, it's refined, simple sugars found in sweetened beverages, juices, candy, baked goods, ready-to-eat cereals, syrups, and many condiments. These types of foods provide quick energy for your body, leading to a rapid increase and decrease in your blood glucose, which then causes your body to crave more or eat another food shortly after.

Foods with refined, simple sugars don't provide much in the way of nutrition. They're typically devoid of vitamins, minerals, or fiber and can work to slow your metabolic rate. Better sources of carbohydrates, which are absorbed more slowly into your bloodstream, include whole grains, fruits, vegetables, and low-fat dairy products. These foods will keep your blood glucose more stable, so you're less vulnerable to cravings.

Giving In — the Right Way

Going cold turkey with the foods you crave will only exacerbate your desire for them and increase the likelihood that you'll overeat that food when faced with it. You have to ask yourself, "Will I really avoid this food that I love forever?" It's not realistic. Therefore, the best action you can take is to indulge in a craving in the healthiest way possible.

Having a healthier version of the food might work sometimes, but not all the time. For example, you could choose frozen yogurt instead of ice cream, which would save you on fat. However, because frozen yogurt has a "health halo," you could end up choosing a large serving of it and eat more calories than if you had a small portion of ice cream. You could actually be more satisfied both physically and mentally with a smaller portion of the full-fat ice cream. Also, when faced with ice cream, you could be prone to also choose a larger portion because you tell yourself "you never eat it and you deserve it." This situation is lose-lose.

To give into cravings the right way, try these methods:

✔ **Have the real food on occasion and plan for it.** Allowing yourself the treat every once in awhile reduces your idealization of it. The frequency of consumption will depend on when you can make room for it in your caloric budget while still achieving a balance of nutrients at each meal.

✔ **Portion out an appropriate serving ahead of time.** Either purchase a pre-portioned food you can't keep in the house in bulk or only buy one serving when you're on-the-go. For example, have a small bag of potato chips or an ounce of chocolate with your sandwich when out to lunch.

✔ **If necessary, pair that food with something nutritious so you're satisfied.** If it's ice cream, you're already getting protein and calcium from it, so that works on its own. If it's a sugary cereal, mix it in with low-fat Greek yogurt for a boost of lean protein that will help slow the absorption of sugar into your bloodstream.

✔ **Remember to savor the food.** If you eat it mindlessly, you won't appreciate it and reap as much satisfaction from having it.

Chapter 17

Ten Metabolism Myths Dispelled

In This Chapter

▶ Identifying what's untrue about your metabolism and weight

▶ Dispelling these myths so you can start off on a healthy track

Do you believe that the fewer calories you eat, the more weight you'll lose? Or are you the type to avoid eating fat because you think it'll go straight to your hips? You may be sabotaging your best efforts at boosting your metabolism and losing weight by holding these myths as gospel because, in many cases, the exact opposite is true.

Throughout your life, you develop eating habits and beliefs that become natural to you, and you stop questioning their validity. At one time, a specific restrictive diet or regimen may have worked to help you lose weight, so you think that because it's not working now, something must be wrong with *you* or your metabolism, not necessarily the nature of the advice. Yes, slow metabolism has become a popular scapegoat.

This chapter can be your cautionary metabolism tale. It'll help you understand why certain myths have been detrimental to your health and your ability to lose weight. It can be a jumping-off point for you to start being a more educated consumer when it comes to food marketing and the media. Instead of following advice blindly, find out the science behind what you hear and gather evidence about how it can be helpful — or not. Knowledge can give you solid footing down a path towards a healthier you.

"I have a slow metabolism, therefore I'll always be overweight"

It's true that your metabolic rate is partly genetic. It's also affected by your age and sex, which are factors beyond your control. But guess what? Your metabolic rate is also affected by your diet, body composition, and activity level, which are all at your fingertips for you to manipulate. Just because you feel like you've been dealt a poor hand with your genes doesn't mean you can't swap out some cards and live better.

When you have this doomed-genes mentality, you think taking steps is useless. But if you're not moving forward, you're really moving backward, and you're making it more and more difficult to lose weight and feel good about yourself. Start small with your goals and focus on three steps to start:

- ✔ Learn the number of calories your body needs (Chapter 3).
- ✔ Start incorporating metabolism-boosting foods (Chapter 5).
- ✔ Think about what activity would realistically fit into your lifestyle (Chapter 11).

No step is too small to take. Most importantly, believe in yourself — you do have the power to make changes to your metabolism.

"If I eat fewer and fewer calories, I'll lose weight"

Weight loss is only about calories in versus calories out, isn't it? Nope! Don't get me wrong, that sure is a big part of the equation. But eat too little or exercise too much, and your weight loss may come to a halt.

All the processes going on in your body require calories, even when you're not moving around. Calories fuel organ function like your heartbeat, breathing, and digestion. If you eat too little to support these functions, your metabolic rate will slow, and your body will stop burning off the calories you eat as effectively.

"Cleanses are the best way to jump-start your metabolism"

Because your metabolism is the method by which your body processes nutrients and uses them for energy, restrictive cleanses actually promote the opposite. Whatever type of cleanse you're referring to, you're likely getting too few calories (see preceding section), and if you're doing a cleanse for a long time, your body will be deprived of nutrients and, therefore, will slow your metabolism down. Plus, your body already has natural detoxification organs built in, such as your kidneys and liver, to filter substances from your blood.

Anecdotally, I often hear people say they experience more energy when doing a cleanse. Think about the fact that you're also cutting down on foods that may slow you down, such as saturated fats and sodium. And because you're depriving yourself, you could be more likely to give in to cravings the minute your cleanse is over.

Instead of a juice cleanse or a fast, try to add more fiber into your diet and complement that with lots of water. A "natural detox" program like that is much cheaper.

"If I work out on an empty stomach, I'll burn more fat"

While this myth does make sense from a scientific standpoint, logistically it doesn't necessarily result in weight loss. The science-y part of it is this: Because you're not eating, your muscles don't have carbohydrates to use for energy, so they turn to fat as their fuel. But that's probably fat located within your muscles, which really doesn't do much for losing overall fat mass in your body. An extremely vigorous training regimen would be required to target your overall fat mass — which you likely wouldn't achieve without eating a snack before, right? Without a snack you'd be fatigued and hungry, and your endurance would go down the drain, sabotaging the whole effort.

Take a tip from athletes who fuel up with balanced meals before and after they workout. Before exercising, choose

- ✔ Whole grain starches and fruits for energy.
- ✔ Lean proteins for muscle strength.
- ✔ Small amounts of heart-healthy fats to keep you satisfied.
- ✔ Substantial amounts of water so you stay hydrated.

As long as you're meeting the goals for amounts of both cardio and strength training in Chapter 11, and you're choosing metabolism-boosting snacks, you'll be burning calories, including those from fat, while keeping that pep in your step.

"Eating fat will make me fat"

Although there are many reasons to reduce your fat intake, bear in mind that anything you eat in excess of what your body needs get stored as fat — whether it's carbohydrates, protein, fat, or ice cream sandwiches. Your body requires fat to do many functions, including creating hormones that help you sense your physical hunger cues. So, getting too little fat can actually result in overeating later on.

You need to get about 20–35 percent of your total calories from fat. To fit within that allowance, choose fats that are unsaturated for your heart's sake:

- **Monounsaturated fats:** Olive oil, canola oil, avocado, nuts, seeds
- **Polyunsaturated fats:** Vegetable oils like corn and sunflower oil, nuts, seeds
- **Omega-3 fatty acids:** Flaxseed, walnuts, and coldwater fish like salmon

"Taking supplements will help me burn fat and lose weight for good"

If your personal trainer or nutritionist is trying to sell you lots of supplements, run — don't walk — out the door. It means they're not focused on helping you make changes for the long term. Supplements may work temporarily by blocking absorption of fat (and healthful nutrients along with it) or manipulating your hormones, but these methods aren't sustainable and can be bad for your health. Instead, focus on a balanced diet and exercise — they may not sound as exciting or convenient, but they're certainly more effective at helping you keep weight off for life.

Always consult with a physician before taking any supplements, because they may interfere with your medication or underlying medical condition.

"If I eat after 8 p.m., I'll gain weight"

You do want to be careful what you eat close to bedtime for a good night's sleep (see Chapter 6), but there's no late-night eating fairy dictating that all calories consumed after 8 p.m. get stored as fat. If you think eating at night is sabotaging your best efforts, ask yourself these questions:

- Am I skipping meals during the day?
- Am I restricting myself too much at each meal?
- Am I mindlessly eating during the day?
- Am I eating at night to help deal with emotions like stress or boredom?

If you answered yes to one or more of these questions, you may be prone to eating more than your body needs later in the evening. That's common, but research repeatedly shows the total amount that you eat and how you spread your calories throughout the day matters more.

"I indulged tonight, so tomorrow I have to hit the gym to make up for it"

You don't need to sweat to burn off the calories of your friend's birthday dinner and drinks. Increasing the activity that you do day to day, such as going for a walk during your lunch break or even fidgeting at your desk at work, burns calories and counts towards your metabolic rate.

To help you remember that being active doesn't mean being a slave to an expensive gym membership, here are some examples of non-exercise activities and the calories they help you burn per hour:

- ✔ **Fidgeting:** 120 calories
- ✔ **Bowling:** 225 calories
- ✔ **Mowing the lawn:** 335 calories
- ✔ **Gardening:** 350 calories

"Some foods, like celery, have negative calories"

I remember my high school health teacher telling us this one, and all the weight-conscious girls' ears perking up. This myth came about because of the fact that your body burns a certain amount of calories to chew and digest foods. The idea is that it takes more calories to eat celery than celery contains.

You won't be able to put your body in a negative calorie balance by eating "negative-calorie" foods like celery, zucchini, cucumber, grapefruit, lemon, broccoli, or lettuce. The amount of calories burned through chewing and digesting is miniscule, unfortunately. However, you should still eat these foods because they're still relatively low-calorie, are chock-full of fiber, vitamins, and minerals, and are good for health.

The only truly natural "zero calorie" food is water. Substituting it for beverages in your diet that are sugary can save you a lot of calories and help you lose weight.

"She's thinner than 1 am, so she must have a faster metabolism"

The more you weigh, the more calories you burn off. So, technically, someone thinner has a *slower* metabolic rate.

As you lose weight, you need fewer and fewer calories to sustain your weight loss. You can keep your metabolism high throughout the process of weight loss by manipulating what you eat and how much you burn through exercise. That way, you're more likely to keep that weight off and keep that furnace burning, even when you turn into the thinner person.

Index

• **E** •

• **N** •

• S •

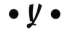

Apple & Mac

iPad For Dummies,
5th Edition
978-1-118-49823-1

iPhone 5 For Dummies,
6th Edition
978-1-118-35201-4

MacBook For Dummies,
4th Edition
978-1-118-20920-2

OS X Mountain Lion
For Dummies
978-1-118-39418-2

Blogging & Social Media

Facebook For Dummies,
4th Edition
978-1-118-09562-1

Mom Blogging
For Dummies
978-1-118-03843-7

Pinterest For Dummies
978-1-118-32800-2

WordPress For Dummies,
5th Edition
978-1-118-38318-6

Business

Commodities For Dummies,
2nd Edition
978-1-118-01687-9

Investing For Dummies,
6th Edition
978-0-470-90545-6

Personal Finance
For Dummies,
7th Edition
978-1-118-11785-9

QuickBooks 2013
For Dummies
978-1-118-35641-8

Small Business Marketing Kit
For Dummies,
3rd Edition
978-1-118-31183-7

Careers

Job Interviews
For Dummies,
4th Edition
978-1-118-11290-8

Job Searching with
Social Media
For Dummies
978-0-470-93072-4

Personal Branding
For Dummies
978-1-118-11792-7

Resumes For Dummies,
6th Edition
978-0-470-87361-8

Success as a Mediator
For Dummies
978-1-118-07862-4

Diet & Nutrition

Belly Fat Diet For Dummies
978-1-118-34585-6

Eating Clean For Dummies
978-1-118-00013-7

Nutrition For Dummies,
5th Edition
978-0-470-93231-5

Digital Photography

Digital Photography
For Dummies,
7th Edition
978-1-118-09203-3

Digital SLR Cameras &
Photography For Dummies,
4th Edition
978-1-118-14489-3

Photoshop Elements 11
For Dummies
978-1-118-40821-6

Gardening

Herb Gardening
For Dummies,
2nd Edition
978-0-470-61778-6

Vegetable Gardening
For Dummies,
2nd Edition
978-0-470-49870-5

Health

Anti-Inflammation Diet
For Dummies
978-1-118-02381-5

Diabetes For Dummies,
3rd Edition
978-0-470-27086-8

Living Paleo For Dummies
978-1-118-29405-5

Hobbies

Beekeeping
For Dummies
978-0-470-43065-1

eBay For Dummies,
7th Edition
978-1-118-09806-6

Raising Chickens
For Dummies
978-0-470-46544-8

Wine For Dummies,
5th Edition
978-1-118-28872-6

Writing Young Adult Fiction
For Dummies
978-0-470-94954-2

Language &
Foreign Language

500 Spanish Verbs
For Dummies
978-1-118-02382-2

English Grammar
For Dummies,
2nd Edition
978-0-470-54664-2

French All-in One
For Dummies
978-1-118-22815-9

German Essentials
For Dummies
978-1-118-18422-6

Italian For Dummies
2nd Edition
978-1-118-00465-4

 Available in print and e-book formats.

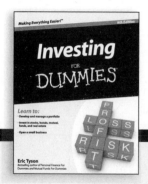 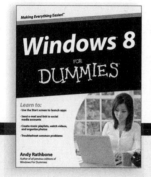 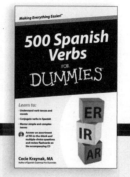 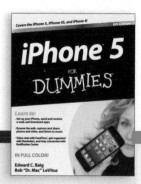

Math & Science

Algebra I For Dummies,
2nd Edition
978-0-470-55964-2

Anatomy and Physiology
For Dummies,
2nd Edition
978-0-470-92326-9

Astronomy For Dummies,
3rd Edition
978-1-118-37697-3

Biology For Dummies,
2nd Edition
978-0-470-59875-7

Chemistry For Dummies,
2nd Edition
978-1-1180-0730-3

Pre-Algebra Essentials
For Dummies
978-0-470-61838-7

Microsoft Office

Excel 2013 For Dummies
978-1-118-51012-4

Office 2013 All-in-One
For Dummies
978-1-118-51636-2

PowerPoint 2013
For Dummies
978-1-118-50253-2

Word 2013 For Dummies
978-1-118-49123-2

Music

Blues Harmonica
For Dummies
978-1-118-25269-7

Guitar For Dummies,
3rd Edition
978-1-118-11554-1

iPod & iTunes
For Dummies,
10th Edition
978-1-118-50864-0

Programming

Android Application
Development For
Dummies, 2nd Edition
978-1-118-38710-8

iOS 6 Application
Development For Dummies
978-1-118-50880-0

Java For Dummies,
5th Edition
978-0-470-37173-2

Religion & Inspiration

The Bible For Dummies
978-0-7645-5296-0

Buddhism For Dummies,
2nd Edition
978-1-118-02379-2

Catholicism For Dummies,
2nd Edition
978-1-118-07778-8

Self-Help & Relationships

Bipolar Disorder
For Dummies,
2nd Edition
978-1-118-33882-7

Meditation For Dummies,
3rd Edition
978-1-118-29144-3

Seniors

Computers For Seniors
For Dummies,
3rd Edition
978-1-118-11553-4

iPad For Seniors
For Dummies,
5th Edition
978-1-118-49708-1

Social Security
For Dummies
978-1-118-20573-0

Smartphones & Tablets

Android Phones
For Dummies
978-1-118-16952-0

Kindle Fire HD
For Dummies
978-1-118-42223-6

NOOK HD For Dummies,
Portable Edition
978-1-118-39498-4

Surface For Dummies
978-1-118-49634-3

Test Prep

ACT For Dummies,
5th Edition
978-1-118-01259-8

ASVAB For Dummies,
3rd Edition
978-0-470-63760-9

GRE For Dummies,
7th Edition
978-0-470-88921-3

Officer Candidate Tests,
For Dummies
978-0-470-59876-4

Physician's Assistant Exam
For Dummies
978-1-118-11556-5

Series 7 Exam
For Dummies
978-0-470-09932-2

Windows 8

Windows 8 For Dummies
978-1-118-13461-0

Windows 8 For Dummies,
Book + DVD Bundle
978-1-118-27167-4

Windows 8 All-in-One
For Dummies
978-1-118-11920-4

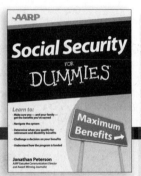 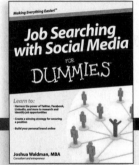 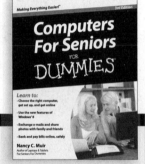 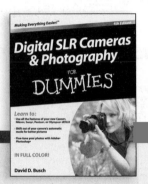

Available in print and e-book formats.

Take Dummies with you everywhere you go!

Whether you're excited about e-books, want more from the web, must have your mobile apps, or swept up in social media, Dummies makes everything easier .

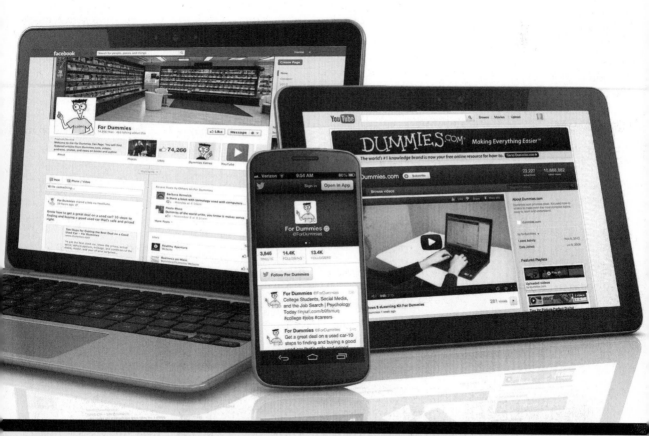

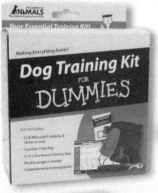
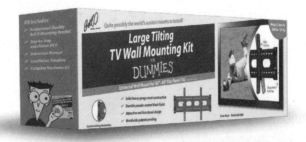
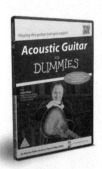
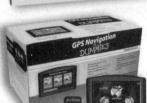
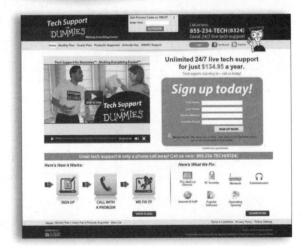
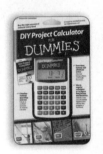
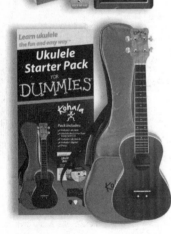
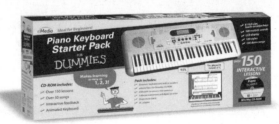
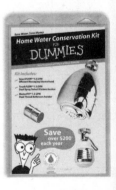